NCLEX Review

The NCLEX Trainer: Content Review of 5 Key Topics, 500+ Specific Practice Questions & Rationales, and Strategies for Test Success

Eva Regan

Contents

Pharmacology

Cardiovascular System

The Respiratory System

Gastrointestinal Disorders

Fluids and Electrolytes

The trademarks that are used are without any consent, and the publication of the trademark is without permission or backing by the trademark owner. All trademarks and brands within this book are for clarifying purposes only and are the owned by the owners themselves, not affiliated with this document.

This book is not intended as a substitute for the medical advice of physicians. The reader should regularly consult a physician in matters relating to his/her health and particularly with respect to any symptoms that may require diagnosis or medical attention.

NCLEX ® holds no affiliation with this product. NCLEX ® is a registered trademark of the National Council of State Boards of Nursing, INC.

Pharmacology

Section 1: Introduction to Pharmacology

Pharmacology is the branch of medicine concerned with the science of drug action on biological systems. As a licensed nurse, one of your main responsibilities is to administer medication to your clients. When administering medication, whether man-made or natural, a nurse should always know how a medication acts in the body, what the safe administration guidelines for that medication are, as well as understand the risks and implications associated with medication administration. When applying their knowledge of pharmacology, nurses must not only know how to safely administer medication but are at times also required to instruct their client or their client's family on the safe administration of medication. Because of this, it is crucial to have a solid understanding of pharmacology and its application within nursing practice.

For test takers, pharmacology is one of the most difficult topics to master. This is because new medications are constantly emerging and there are already an enormous amount of available medications in common use. It is therefore important to spend enough time reviewing pharmacology in your preparation for the NCLEX. In the exam, you may be presented with a medication that you are not familiar with. In this case you will need to be able to make an educated guess. In this guide, you will be provided with strategies and guidelines that you can apply in order to make an educated guess.

3

The guide begins with an outline of the topics and key facts that you need to remember for the exam. The list of subtopics can be seen on the contents page. This is all presented with helpful notes, tips, and cautions. In Section 3 of this guide you can apply and test your knowledge with over 100 topic-specific practice questions. All answers to the questions are given with detailed rationales to further your knowledge and understanding of the topic.

Remember that ambition is the first step to success. The second step is action – hard work and determination. Purchasing this guide is an indication of your ambition, now it's time to get to work!

Best wishes,

Eva Regan

Section 2: Pharmacology Study Checklist

1. <u>Three Areas of Pharmacology</u>

It's important to remember that pharmacology includes three areas:

Pharmacokinetics:

This is the study of how medications are absorbed, metabolized, distributed and excreted by the body.

Pharmacokinetics is particularly relevant when it comes to clients with renal or liver disease or elderly clients who frequently encounter difficulties when it comes to metabolizing and excreting medications.

Pharmacodynamics:

This is the study of how medications are used by the body.

Pharmacotherapeutics:

This is the study of how the client responds to the drug.

2. <u>Pharmacology In Nursing Practice</u>

In nursing practice, nurses are expected to apply their

knowledge of pharmacology in order to:

- Recognize common uses, side effects, and adverse effects of their client's medication.
- Meet the learning needs of their client.
- Challenge medication errors.

Test takers need to remember the medication classifications commonly used in medical and surgical settings and their effects on the body:

- **Antacids:** Antacids reduce hydrochloric acid in the stomach. Constipation is a common side effect of calcium- and aluminum-based antacids. Diarrhea is a common side effect of magnesium-based antacids.

- **Anti-infectives:** Anti-infectives are used to treat infections. A common side effect includes GI upset.

- **Antianemics:** Antianemics increase red blood cell production by increasing the amount of haemoglobin in the blood or number of red blood cells. B12, iron, and Epogen (erythropoetin) are all examples of antianemics.

- **Anticholinergics:** Anticholinergics are used to induce dryness in mucous membranes which causes a decrease in oral secretions. Anticholinergics such as atropine are often administered prior to operations.

- **Anticoagulants:** Anticoagulants prevent the coagulation, i.e. clotting of blood. They achieve this by preventing platelet aggregation or by decreasing vitamin K levels and blocking the clotting chain.

- **Anticonvulsants:** Anticonvulsants are used in the treatment of seizure disorder and of bipolar disorder. Phenobarbital, phenytoin (Dilantin), and lorazepam (Ativan) are all medications in this category.

- **Antidiarrheals:** Antidiarrheals reduce water content in the intestinal tract and lower gastric motility. Bloating and gas are common side effects.

- **Antihistamines:** Antihistamines block the release of histamine during allergic reactions. Signs of dry mouth, drowsiness, and sedation are common side effects caused by antihistamines.

- **Antihypertensives:** Antihypertensives lower blood pressure as well as increase blood flow to the myocardium. Orthostatic hypotension is a common side effect. Other side effects may arise which are specific to types of antihypertensive prescribed.

- **Antipyretics:** Antipyretics reduce fever.

- **Bronchodilators:** Bronchodilators dilate large air passages. They are commonly prescribed for clients who suffer from asthma and chronic obstructive lung disease. Tachycardia is a common side effect.

- **Diuretics:** Diuretics decrease the absorption of water and sodium from the loop of Henle (loop diuretics) or inhibit antidiuretic hormone (potassium-sparing diuretics). Hypokalemia is a side effect of non-potassium-sparing diuretics.

- **Laxatives:** Laxatives loosen stools and increase bowel movements. Types of laxatives include cathartics, fiber, lubricants, stimulants, and stool softeners.

- **Miotics:** Miotics onstrict the pupil. Miotics such as pilocarpine HCl are used to treat clients with glaucoma.

- **Mydriatics:** Mydriatics dilate the pupils. They are used to treat clients with cataracts.

- **Narcotic analgesics:** Narcotic analgesics are drugs that relieve moderate to severe pain. A common side effect is numbness. They can also induce a state of unconsciousness. Opioids (morphine and codeine), synthetic opioids (meperidine), and NSAIDs (ketorolac) are all medications in this category.

3. Administering Medications

The 'Seven Rights' of Administering Medication is a checklist that needs to be memorized by every nursing student and nurse. They include five rights of drug administration and two rights that stem from the Patient's Bill of Rights. The seven rights must be used every time a client is administered a medication by a nurse.

The 'Seven Rights' of Patient Medication include:

4. The Right Medication
5. The Right Patient;
6. The Right Dose;

7. The Right Time;
8. The Right Route;
9. The Right Reason
10. The Right Documentation.

The Right Medication: The nurse should check both the generic and trade names with the physician's order in order to ensure that the correct medication is administered. In the case that the client's diagnosis does not match the drug category, the nurse must investigate the ordered medication.

The Right Patient: The nurse should take steps to identify the client by checking the identification band and by asking the client to state his name.

The Right Dose: The nurse must know common dosages for both adults and children.

The Right Time: The nurse is expected administer the medication either 30 minutes before or 30 minutes after the assigned time.

The Right Route: The physician orders the prescribed route of administration. This should be followed provided it complies with formulary guidelines.

The Right Reason / Right to Refuse Treatment: The client has the right to refuse treatment, which includes medications, if a client refuses medication, the nurse should determine the reasons for refusal.

The Right Documentation: The nurse must always document treatment given to the client. Documentation must be done promptly and accurately to ensure that medication administration is not duplicated.

4. Time-Released Drugs

Medication that contains one of the abbreviations below are 'time-released drugs.' This means they should under no circumstances be opened, dissolved or crushed before being administered to the client.

- Contin = Continuous action
- CR = Continuous release
- Dur = Duration
- LA = Long acting
- SA = Sustained action
- SR = Sustained release

Enteric-coated tablets and caplets: These are medications that are coated with a thick shell. This allows for the medication to be absorbed more slowly and prevents the medication from being absorbed in the upper GI tract.

Spansules: These are capsules that contain time-released beads that are released slowly. If the client cannot swallow a time-released medication, then the physician should be notified in order to obtain a different preparation for the client. The nurse should never alter the preparation.

5. Drug Schedules

Nurses and nursing students must also know the various drug schedules. This will no doubt crop up in questions relating to safety.

- **Schedule I:** Not currently accepted for medical use and are for research use only (for example, LSD). These are drugs with high potential for abuse.

- **Schedule II:** These drugs have a high potential for abuse and therefore require a written prescription for each refill. Examples of drugs under this schedule narcotics, stimulants and barbiturates for example. No telephone renewals are allowed.

- **Schedule III:** These require a new prescription after six months or five refills. Examples of drugs under this schedule include codeine, steroids, and antidepressants. Can be ordered by telephone.

- **Schedule IV:** These require a new prescription after six months, e.g. benzodiazepines.

- **Schedule V:** These can be dispensed as any other prescription or without prescription (if state law allows). Examples of drugs under this schedule include antidiarrheals and antitussives.

6. <u>Pregnancy Categories</u>

One can never say whether it is 100% safe to use a medication on a pregnant client. Because of this, medications are split up into categories of safety by risk level. There are certain categories of medication a pregnant client must avoid and it is important for a nurse to be aware of these categories. Knowledge of these categories is also likely to be tested on the NCLEX exam

- **Category A:** The safest drugs to take during pregnancy. No risk to fetus.

- **Category B:** Insufficient data to use in pregnancy. Studies for fetal effects in animals have found no risks but no adequate studies on pregnant women are available.

- **Category C:** Potential benefits of medication may warrant use of this medication on pregnant women despite potential risks.

- **Category D:** Risk to fetus exists, but potential benefits of the medication could outweigh the probable risks.

- **Category X:** There is positive evidence of human fetal risk. Avoid use of these medications in pregnancy or in those who may become pregnant. Potential risks to the fetus outweigh the potential benefits.

7. Herbal Remedies

Although herbals are not considered to be medications by some, they do however have medicinal properties. On the NCLEX exam, herbals are included as a subtopic under pharmacology. The following is a list of the most common herbals used and the necessary guidelines a nurse or nursing student should be aware of.

Echinacea:

- Uses: To treat fevers, colds and urinary tract infections.
- Reactions: This herbal can potentially interfere with methotrexate, ketoconazole and immunosuppressive agents.

Feverfew:

- Uses: To treat and prevent migraines, arthritis, and fever.
- Reactions: This herbal should not be taken in conjunction with aspirin, NSAIDs, Coumadin, thrombolytics, or antiplatelet medications. This is because it will prolong the bleeding time.

Ginkgo:

- Uses: This herbal improves memory and can be used to treat depression. Ginkgo also promotes peripheral circulation.
- Reactions: This herbal should not be taken with MAO inhibitors, anticoagulants, or antiplatelets. This is because it increases the bleeding time in clients taking NSAIDs, cephalosporins, and valproic acid. Ginkgo should also be avoided by clients with seizure disorders because it can exacerbate seizure activity.

Ginseng:

- Uses: Ginseng is used as an anti-inflammatory. This herbal enhances the immune system, improves mental and physical abilities and has estrogen effects.
- Reactions: Ginseng decreases the effects of anticoagulants and NSAIDs. This herbal must be avoided by clients taking corticosteroids. This is because ginseng and corticosteroids when taken in combination can result in extremely high levels of corticosteroids. High doses cause liver problems. Clients with hypertension and bipolar disorder must be cautioned regarding the use of ginseng because it can interfere with medications used to treat these disorders.

Kava-kava:

- Uses: Kava-kava is used to treat insomnia as well as mild muscle aches and pains.
- Reactions: This herbal increases the effects of central nervous system (CNS) suppressants and decreases those of levodopa. The use of kava-kava can also increase the effect of MAOIs and cause liver damage.

Ma Huang:

- Uses: Ma Huang is used for weight loss and to increase energy levels. It is also used to treat asthma and hay fever.
- Reactions: This herbal increases the effect of MAOIs, cardiac glycosides, theophylline, and sympathomimetics.

St. John's Wort:

- Uses: This herbal is used to treat mild to moderate depression.
- Reactions: St. John's Wort increases adverse CNS effects when used with alcohol or antidepressant medications.

8. <u>Understanding and Knowing How to Identify Drugs</u>

Firstly, it is important to understand that drugs have several names:

- **The chemical name:** This is usually a number or letter that is indicative of the chemical makeup of the medication. This name is not of much value to a practicing nurse.
- **The generic name:** This is the name given to the drug by the company that developed it. It is much safer for a nurse to remember this name because the generic name always remains the same.
- **The trade name:** once a drug has been released to the market for around four years, a trade-named

medication can be released by another company. While the generic name will stay the same, the trade name will be different.

If you can, it is best to remember both the trade and the generic name of a drug. On the exam, the generic name will be given and the trade name may at times be included for further clarification.

Roughly 80% of generic drugs within the same category have common syllables. Recognizing and identifying these commonalities will significantly help you study for the NCLEX. The following categories in this section are designed to help you recognize these commonalities in the drug names. This will help you to quickly identify a specific drug and thereby their drug category.

1. _Angiotensin-Converting Enzyme (ACE) Inhibitors_
- **Uses:** These Antihypertensives are used in the treatment of both primary and secondary hypertensions.
- **Reactions:** These drugs inhibit conversion of angiotensin I to angiotensin II.
- **Syllable:** PRIL.

You will notice that all the generic names include the syllable 'pril'. If you see the syllable 'pril', this is an indication that the medication is an ACE enzyme inhibitor. Examples include:

Benazepril (Lotensin), lisinopril (Zestril), captopril (Capoten), enalapril (Vasotec), fosinopril (Monopril), moexipril (Univas), quinapril (Acupril), ramipril (Altace). On top of identifying an ACE inhibitor, it is important that you know and remember the potential side effects and adverse reactions of ACE enzyme inhibitors when working with the drug.

Side effects and adverse reactions associated with ACE inhibitors include:

- Angioedema
- Hacking cough
- Hypotension
- Nausea and/or vomiting
- Rashes

Nursing considerations to know and use when working with ACE inhibitors:

- Monitor the electrolyte levels
- Monitor the potassium and creatinine levels
- Monitor the vital signs frequently
- Monitor the white blood cell count

2. *Angiotensin Receptor Blockers*
- **Uses:** Angiotensin receptor blockers are used to treat primary or secondary hypertension. These drugs are used to treat clients who complain of coughing that can be linked ot the use of ACE inhibitors.
- **Reactions:** These drugs block vasoconstrictor- and aldosterone-secreting angiotensin II.

- **Syllable:** SARTAN.

When you see the syllable 'sartan', you'll know that the drug is an angiotensin receptor blocker. Examples include: Candesartan (Altacand), Losartan (Cozaar), Valsartan (Diovan), and Telmisartan (Micardis).

Side effects and adverse reactions associated with angiotensin receptor blockers include:

- Cough
- Depression
- Diarrhea
- Dizziness
- Impotence
- Insomnia
- Muscle cramps
- Nausea/vomiting
- Neutropenia

Nursing interventions to know and use when working with clients that are taking angiotensin receptor blocker agents:

- Instruct the client to check edema in feet and legs daily.
- Monitor blood pressure.
- Monitor BUN.
- Monitor creatinine.
- Monitor electrolytes.
- Monitor hydration status.

3. *Anticoagulants*
- **Uses:** Anticoagulant drugs are used to treat deep-vein myocardial infarction, pulmonary emboli, thrombosis and thrombolytic disease. These medications are also used after coronary artery bypass surgery and for other conditions, such as those requiring anticoagulation.
- **Reactions:** These drugs thin the blood and are therefore used to treat clotting disorders.
- **Syllable:** PARIN.

When you see the syllable 'parin', you'll know that the drug is a anticoagulant. Examples include: Dalteparin sodium (Fragmin), Enoxaparin Sodium (Lovenox), and Heparin Sodium (Hepalean).

Side effects and adverse reactions associated with anticoagulant drugs include:

- Alopecia
- Bleeding
- Dermatitis
- Diarrhea
- Fever
- Hematuria
- Pruritus
- Stomatitis

Nursing interventions to know and use when working with clients that are taking anticoagulant agents:

- Check blood studies (hematocrit and occult blood in stool) every three months
- Monitor for signs of bleeding
- Monitor for signs of infection
- Monitor platelet count
- Perform a PTT check on clients taking **Heparin Sodium** (Hepalean) to evaluate the bleeding time (therapeutic levels are 1.5–2.0 times the control)
- No specific bleeding time is done for **Enoxaparin Sodium** (Lovenox), but platelet levels must be checked for thrombocytopenia

4. _Anti-Infectives (Aminoglycosides)_
- **Uses:** These drugs are used to either kill an infectious agent or inhibit it from spreading.
- **Reactions:** Anti-infective drugs interfere with the protein synthesis of bacteria, thereby causing the bacteria to die. Anti-infectives are active against some gram-positive organisms and against most aerobic gram-negative bacteria.
- **Note:** Anti-infectives are often used in the treatment of super-infections, e.g. methicillin-resistant staphylococcus aureus (MRSA). The symptoms of clients with MRSA include: cough, diarrhea, fever, malaise, pain, perineal itching, redness, stomatitis and swelling.
- **Syllable:** CIN or MYCIN.

Anti-infectives include bactericidals and bacteriostatics. These drugs end with the syllable 'cin' and many of them end in 'mycin.' Examples include: Gentamicin (Garamycin, Alcomicin, Genoptic), kanamycin (Kantrex), neomycin (Mycifradin), streptomycin (Streptomycin), tobramycin

(Tobrex, Nebcin), amikacin (Amikin).

Side effects and adverse reactions associated with anti-infectives include:

- Blood dyscrasias
- Hypotension
- Nephrotoxicity
- Ototoxicity
- Rash
- Seizures

Nursing interventions to know and use when working with clients that are taking anti-infectives:

- Obtain history of allergies
- Instruct the client to report any chances in renal function, i.e. urinary elimination, or in hearing. (This is because these drugs can be toxic to the auditory nerve and to the kidney)
- Monitor for therapeutic levels
- Monitor for signs of nephrotoxicity
- Monitor for signs of ototoxicity
- Monitor a patent IV site
- Monitor intake and output
- Monitor peak and through levels
- Monitor vital signs during intravenous infusion

5. *Antivirals*
- **Uses:** Antivirals are used for their antiviral properties. Clients that suffer from AIDS are often treated with either one or a combination of antiviral. Antiviral

drugs are also used in the treatment of HSV-1 and HSV-2, chickenpox, shingles, fever blisters, encephalitis, cytomegalovirus (CMV), and respiratory syncytial virus (RSV).
- **Reactions:** Antivirals inhibit enzymes with a virus, thereby inhibiting viral growth.
- **Syllable:** VIR.

When you see the syllable 'vir', you'll know that the drug is an antiviral. Examples include: Acyclovir (Zovirax), Abacavir (Ziagen), Cidofovir (Vistide), Indinavir (Crixivan), Ritonavir (Norvir), and Saquinovir (Invirase, Fortovase).

Side effects and adverse reactions associated with antivirals include:

- Diarrhea
- Nausea
- Oliguria
- Proteinuria
- Vaginitis
- Vomiting
- Central nervous side effects are also possible although these are less common:
  - Tremors
  - Confusion
  - Seizures
  - Severe/sudden anemia

Nursing interventions to know and use when working with clients that are taking antiviral drugs:

- Be watchful for signs of infection

- Instruct the client to report any signs of a rash as this can be indicative of an allergic reaction
- Monitor bowel pattern before and during treatment
- Monitor liver profile

Monitor the creatinine level frequently

6. _Benzodiazepines (Anticonvulsants/Antianxiety) drugs_
- **Uses:** Benzodiazepines are used for their anti-anxiety or anti-convulsant effects, e.g. to reduce anxiety, to induce relaxation, to treat or prevent seizures and panic disorders, among other things.
- **Syllable:** PAM, PATE, or LAM.

When trying to identify benzodiazepines, it is useful to remember that while some contain the syllable 'pam', others contain 'pate' or 'lam'. All benzodiazepines however will contain 'azo' or 'aze'. Examples include Clonazepam (Klonopin), diazepam (Valium), chlordiazepoxide (Librium), lorazepam (Ativan), flurazepam (Dalmane)

Side effects and adverse reactions associated with benzodiazepines include:

- Ataxia
- Bradycardia
- Constipation
- Depression
- Diplopia
- Drowsiness
- Hypotension
- Incontinence

- Lethargy
- Nausea/vomiting
- Nystagmus
- Rash
- Respiratory depression
- Restlessness
- Slurred speech
- Urinary retention
- Urticaria

Nursing interventions to know and use when working with benzodiazepines:

- Monitor respirations
- Monitor liver function
- Monitor kidney function
- Monitor bone marrow function
- Monitor for signs of chemical abuse

7. *Beta Adrenergic Blockers*
- **Uses:** These drugs help lower blood pressure, pulse rate, and cardiac output. Beta adrenergic blockers are also used in the treatment of migraines and other vascular headaches. Certain preparations of this drug can also be used in the treatment of glaucoma and to prevent myocardial infarctions.
- **Reactions:** Beta adrenergic blockers act by blocking the sympathetic vasomotor response.
- **Syllable:** OLOL.

When you see the syllable 'olol', you'll know that the drug is a beta blocker. Examples include Acebutolol (Monitan,

Rhotral, Sectral), Atenolol (Tenormin, Apo-Atenol, Nova-Atenol), Carvedilol (Coerg), Esmolol (Brevibloc) and Toprol-XL (Metoprolol). On top of being able to identify beta adrenergic blockers, nurses and nurse students must also know the potential side effects and adverse effects.

Side effects and adverse reactions associated with beta adrenergic blockers include:

- Bradycardia
- Diarrhea
- Nausea and/or vomiting
- Orthostatic hypertension
- May mask hypoglycemic symptoms

Nursing interventions to know and use when working with clients that are taking beta adrenergic blockers:

- Teach the client to:
  - Taper off the medication
  - Rise slowly
  - Report bradycardia, dizziness, confusion, depression or any signs of fever
- Monitor the client's blood pressure, heart rate, and rhythm
- Monitor the client for changes in lab values (BUN, creatinine, protein) that indicate nephrotic syndrome
- Monitor the client for signs of edema. The nurse must assess lung sounds for rhonchi and rales.

8. *Cholesterol-Lowering Agents*
- **Uses:** Cholesterol-Lowering Agents are use to reduce cholesterol and triglyceride levels. These drugs are also used decrease the potential for cardiovascular disease and to
- **Note:** Cholesterol-lowering drugs should not be taken with grapefruit juice. They should be taken at night and the client must have undergone liver studies prior to taking cholesterol-lowering agents to determine the presence of liver disease.
- **Syllable:** VASTATIN.
- **Caution:** Do not confuse with 'statin' drugs that are used for their antifungal effects, such as Nystatin.

When you see the syllable 'vastatin', you'll know that the drug is a cholesterol-lowering agent. Examples include: Atorvastatin (Lipitor), fluvastatin (Lescol), lovastatin (Mevacor), pravastatin (Pravachol), simvastatin (Zocar), rosuvastatin (Crestor).

Side effects and adverse reactions associated with cholesterol-lowering drugs include:

- Alopecia
- Dyspepsia
- Headache
- Liver dysfunction
- Myalgia (muscle weakness)
- Rash

Nursing interventions to know and use when working with clients that are taking cholesterol-lowering agents:

- Include a diet low in cholesterol and fat
- Instruct the client to report any unexplained muscle soreness or weakness and cola-colored urine to the physician
- Monitor cholesterol levels
- Monitor for muscle weakness and pain
- Monitor liver profile
- Monitor renal function

9. *Glucocorticoids*

- **Uses:** Glucocorticoids are used to decrease inflammatory responses to allergies and inflammatory diseases, to reduce the possibility of organ plant rejection, and to treat conditions that require suppression of the immune system. These drugs are also used in the treatment of Addison's disease, chronic obstructive pulmonary disease, and immune disorders.

- **Reactions:** Glucocorticoids have anti-allergenic, anti-inflammatory, and anti-stress effects.

- **Note:** Glucocorticoid drugs can cause Cushing's syndrome. Symptoms include buffalo hump, edema, elevated blood glucose levels, hirsutism, moon faces, purple straie, and weight gain.

- **Syllable:** SONE or CORT.

When you see the syllable 'sone' or 'cort', you'll know that the drug is a glucocorticoid. Examples include: Prednisolone (Delta-Cortef, Prednisol, Prednisolone), prednisone (Apo-Prednisone, Deltasone, Meticorten, Orasone, Panasol-S), betamethasone (Celestone, Selestoject, Betnesol), dexamethasone (Decadron, Deronil, Dexon, Mymethasone,

Dalalone), cortisone (Cortone), hydrocortisone (Cortef, Hydrocortone Phosphate, Cortifoam), methylprednisolone (Solu-cortef, Depo-Medrol, Depopred, Medrol, Rep-Pred), triamcinolone (Amcort, Aristocort, Atolone, Kenalog, Triamolone).

Side effects and adverse reactions associated with glucocorticoid drugs include:

- Acne
- Bruising
- Depression
- Depression
- Diarrhea
- Ecchymosis
- Flushing
- Hemorrhage
- Hypertension
- Hypomania
- Insomnia
- Leukocytosis
- Osteoporosis
- Petechiae
- Poor wound healing
- Sweating

Nursing interventions to know and use when working with clients that are taking glucocorticoid drugs:

- Monitor blood pressure
- Monitor for signs of infection
- Monitor glucose levels
- Weigh the client on a daily basis

10. *Histamine 2 Antagonists*

- **Uses:** Histamine 2 antagonist drugs are used to decrease acid production and to treat acid reflux, gastric ulcers, and GERD.
- **Reactions:** These agents inhibit gastric acids by inhibiting histamine 2 release in the gastric parietal cells.
- **Syllable:** TIDINE.

When you see the syllable 'tidine', you'll know that the drug is a histamine 2 antagonist. Examples include: Cimetidine (Tagamet), Famotidine (Pepcid), Nizatidine (Axid), and Rantidine (Zantac).

Side effects and adverse reactions associated with histamine 2 antagonists include:

Confusion

- Agranulocytosis
- Alopecia
- Bradycardia/tachycardia
- Diarrhea
- Galactorrhea
- Gynecomastia
- Psychosis
- Rash
- Seizures

Nursing interventions to know and use when working with clients that are taking histamine 2 antagonist drugs:

- Administer the drugs with meals

- Cimetidine can be prescribed in one large dose at bedtime
- If the client is taking antacids as well as histamine 2 antagonists, make sure the client takes antacids one hour before or after taking these medications
- Monitor the blood urea nitrogen levels
- Sucralfate reduces the effects of histamine 2 receptor blockers

11. *Phenothiazines (Antipsychotic/Antiemetic) drugs*

- **Uses:** Phenotiazines are used as antiemetics, neuroleptics or major tranquilizers. These drugs are used in the treatment of psychosis in clients with schizophrenia. Certain phenothiazine drugs, e.g. Phenergan (promethazine) and Compazine (prochlorperzine), are used to treat nausea and vomiting.
- **Note:** Phenotiazines are irritating to the tissue. Because of this, Z-track method should be used to administer this drug by intramuscular injection. A client who is allergic to this a phenothiazine drug is likely to be allergic to all of them. A client who experiences an allergic reaction, extrapyramidal effects or any more severe reactions needs to be given **Congentin** (benztropine mesylate) or **Benadryl** (hdiphenhydramine hydrochloride).
- **Syllable:** ZINE.

When you see the syllable 'ZINE', you'll know that the drug is a phenothiazine. Examples include: Chlopromazine (Thorazine), prochlorperazine (Compazine), trifluoperazine (Stelazine), promethazine (Phenergan), hydroxyzine

(Vistaril), fluphenazine (Prolixin).

Side effects and adverse reactions associated with phenothiazines include:

- Agranulocytosis
- Drowsiness
- Dry mouth
- Extrapyramidal effects
- Neuroleptic malignant syndrome
- Orthostatic hypotension
- Photosensitivity
- Sedation

Nursing interventions to know and use when working with clients that are taking phenothiazines:

- Be cautious: liquid forms of Fluphenazine (Prolixin) should not be mixed with any beverage containing caffeine, tannates, or pectin due to physical incompatibility
- Monitor liver enzymes
- Monitor renal function
- Protect the client from overexposure to the sun
- Protect the drug from light

12. *Proton Pump Inhibitors*
- **Uses:** Proton pump inhibitors are used to treat indigestion, esophagitis, gastric ulcers, and GERD.
- **Reactions:** These inhibitors inhibit the hydrogen/potassium ATPase enzyme system, thereby suppressing gastric secretion.

- **Syllable:** PRAZOLE.

When you see the syllable 'prazole', you'll know that the drug is a proton pump inhibitor. Examples include: Esomeprazole (Nexium), Lansoprazole (Prevacid), Pantoprazole (Protonix), and Rabeprazole (AciPhex).

Side effects and adverse reactions associated with proton pump inhibitors include:

- Diarrhea
- Flatulence
- Headache
- Hyperglycemia
- Insomnia
- Rash

Nursing interventions to know and use when working with clients that are taking proton pump inhibitors:

- Instruct the client to always take the medication prior to meals
- Monitor liver function
- Use a filter when administering IV pantoprazole – don't crush pantoprazole (Protonix)

To pass the NCLEX, you will need to learn the specific classification of a drug. Remember that learning these classifications will make studying for the pharmacology significantly easier - this is because medications within a certain category share the same commonalities.

When revising for the NCLEX, it is therefore crucial to remember:

- The specific classification of a medication, its actions inside the body, and all associated side effects and adverse effects
- How to safely administer a medication within that specific classification

9. Other Useful Drug Identification Clues:

Below are some other clues helpers that can assist you in identifying drug types:

- **Caine** = Anesthetics (Lidocaine)
- **Cal** = Calciums (Calcimar)
- **Ceph or cef** = Cephalosporins (Cefatazime)
- **Cillin** = Penicillins (Ampicillin)
- **Cycline** = tetracycline (Tetracycline) (Note that Tetracycline should never be given to a pregnant woman or small children)
- **Done** = Opioids (Methodone)
- **Mab** = Monoclonal antibodies (Palivazumab)
- **Phylline** = Bronchodilators (Aminophylline)
- **Stigmine** = Cholinergics (Phyostigmine)

Looking at the similarities and commonalities between medications will help you to identify a certain type of drug, know their side effects and the relevant nursing interventions. This will also help you manage and divide the substantial knowledge that you need to successfully pass the test.

I encourage you to review this section often to ensure you remember all essential facts and information. Do not worry if you don't feel entirely confident yet - start testing yourself on realistic practice questions which you can find in the next section. Go over any questions you get incorrect, working out why, and then improve your knowledge in that specific area.

Section 3: Pharmacology Practice Questions and Rationales

1. While acquiring information about the current medication use of the client, the client tells the nurse that they take the herbal supplement ginkgo to improve mental alertness. The nurse should inform the client to:

a. Avoid any exposure to the sun whilst using ginkgo.

b. Buy only brands with FDA approval.

c. Increase daily intake of vitamin E.

d. Report signs of bleeding or bruising or to the doctor.

Answer D is correct. Ginkgo interacts with many different medications to increase the risk of bleeding. Because of this, bruising or bleeding should be reported to the doctor. Answer A is incorrect, because photosensitivity is not a side effect of ginkgo. The FDA does not regulate herbals and natural products, and therefore Answer B is also incorrect. Lastly, the client does not need to take additional vitamin E, therefore answer C is also incorrect.

2. The client has a prescription for a calcium carbonate compound in order to neutralize stomach acid. The nurse should assess the client for:

a. Diarrhea

b. Constipation

c. Hyperphosphatemia

d. Hypomagnesemia

Answer B is correct. A client using calcium preparations will frequently develop constipation. Answers B, C, and D do not apply in this scenario.

3. Which of the following medications are category X medications and should therefore not be taken by the client during pregnancy?

a. Cefozolin
b. Devonex
c. Levothyroxine
d. Menocycline
e. Tazorac

Answers B, D, and E are correct. Devonex, Minocycline, and Tazorac and are all medications under category X and should therefore not be given during pregnancy because they are teratagenic.

4. Your client is taking alendronate sodium (Fosamax). Which instruction should you give to your client?

a. Remain in an upright position for 30 minutes after taking this medication

b. Take the medication while lying down
c. Force fluids while taking this medication
d. Take the medication together with estrogen

Answer A is correct. This drug causes gastric reflux, so the client should remain upright and take it with only water. Alendronate sodium is a drug used in the treatment of osteoporosis. Alendronate sodium should not be taken while lying down and should not be taken in conjunction with another medication or with estrogen.
Notice: there is a clue in the name of the drug: *fosa*, as in fossils. All the drugs in this category contain the syllable *dronate*.

5. A client is discharged with a prescription for Evista (raloxifene HCl). The nurse should inform the client of which of the following is a side effect of this drug?

a. Urinary frequency
b. Leg cramps
c. Hot flashes
d. Cold extremities

Answer C is correct. Evista is a drug used in the treatment of osteoporosis. The medication has an agonist effect, which binds with estrogen and which can cause hot flashes. The medication does not cause any of the other symptoms and answers A, B, and D are therefore incorrect.
Notice: The E in Evista stands for estrogen. This medication

is in the same category as the chemotherapeutic agent tamoxifene (Novaldex) which is used for breast cancer.

6. The client, an elderly diabetic, is scheduled for a cardiac catheterization. The client has been taking metformin (Glucophage). The nurse should instruct the client to:

a. Take the medication with only water prior to the exam
b. Take the medication as usual prior to the exam
c. Limit protein intake prior to the exam
d. Discontinue the medication prior to the exam

Answer D is correct. This is because Glucophage can cause renal problems. The dye used in cardiac catheterizations is likewise detrimental to the kidneys. After the cardiac catheterizations or until renal function returns, the client may be placed on sliding scale insulin for 48 hours.
Note that B and D are opposites. B is incorrect because the client should stop taking the medication prior to the exam. Answer A is incorrect because taking Glucophage with water is not necessary. And Answer C is likewise incorrect because limiting protein intake prior to the exam has no correlation to the medication.

Notice: The syllable 'phage' (as seen in the syllable 'phage') means eating.

7. The client is taking furosemide (Lasix). Which of the

following laboratory results should be of concern to the nurse?

a. Sodium level of 140
b. Potassium level of 2.5
c. Glucose level of 110
d. Calcium level of 8

Answer B is correct. This is because Furosemide (Lasix) is a loop diuretic.

Notice: Most loop diuretics end in the syllable 'ide'.

8. A client who has just undergone an exploratory laparotomy is admitted to the recovery room. Which of the following medication should be kept nearby?

a. Diphenhydramine (Benadryl)
b. Flumazenil (Romazicon)
c. Naloxone hydrochloride (Narcan)
d. Nitroprusside (Nipride)

Answer C is correct. Answer C is correct because Narcan is the antidote to narcotics. During the postoperative period, narcotics are given to the client. Answer A is also incorrect because Benadryl is an antihistamine. Answer B is incorrect because Romazicon is the antidote for the benzodiazepines. Answer D is incorrect because Nipride is used to lower blood pressure.

9. The client with renal failure has a subscription for erythropoietin (Epogen) which is to be given subcutaneously. The nurse should instruct the client to report which of the following symptoms?

a. Decreased urination
b. Itching
c. Severe headache
d. Slight nausea

Answer C is correct. This is because severe headache can indicate impending seizure activity. It should therefore be immediately reported. Answer A and C are incorrect because a client with renal failure already suffers from itching and decreased urination. Answer D is incorrect because slight nausea is expected when beginning the therapy.

10. A four-year-old client with cystic fibrosis has an order for Viokase pancreatic enzymes to prevent malabsorption. The pancreatic enzyme should be administered:

a. On an empty stomach

b. One hour before meals

c. Two hours after meals

d. With each meal and snack

Answer D is correct. Viokase is a pancreatic enzyme used to facilitate digestion. The enzyme should therefore be given with meals and snacks. Viokase works well in foods such as applesauce. Answers A, B, and C are all incorrect.

11. A 20-year-old client has an order for tetracycline. While teaching the client how to take the medicine, the nurse is told that the client is currently also using Ortho-Novum, an oral contraceptive pill. The nurse should inform the client that:

a. Antibiotics can decrease the effectiveness of oral contraceptives. Because of this, the client should use different type of birth control.

b. Nausea often results from taking oral contraceptives and antibiotics.

c. The oral contraceptives will decrease the effectiveness of the tetracycline.

d. Toxicity can result when taking these two medications together.

Answer A is correct. Taking both antibiotics and oral contraceptives at the same time decreases the effectiveness of the oral contraceptives. The client should therefore be advised to take use a different type of birth control.

12. The nurse is visiting a home health client with osteoporosis who has a new prescription for alendronate (Fosamax). Which instruction should be included in the teaching plan?

a. Avoid rapid movements after taking Fosamax.

b. Don't take any other medications for 30 minutes after taking the Fosamax.

c. Rest in bed for at least half an hour after taking the medication.

d. Take the medication with water only and remain upright for at least 30 minutes after taking the medication.

Answer D is correct. Fosamax should be taken with water only. The client should also remain upright for at least 30 minutes after taking the medication. Answer C is the opposite of Answer D and is therefore incorrect. Answers A and B are not applicable to taking Fosamax and are therefore also incorrect.

13. The client diagnosed with multiple myeloma has a subscription for cyclophosphamide (Cytoxan). The nurse should instruct the client to:

a. "Drink at least eight large glasses of water a day."

b. "Immediately report nausea to the doctor."

c. "Increase the fiber intake in your diet."

d. "Walk for at least 30 minutes a day to prevent calcium loss."

Answer A is correct. The medication can cause hemorrhagic cystitis and because of this, the client should drink at least eight glasses of water a day. Answers B is incorrect as nausea often occurs with chemotherapy. Answers C and D are both not necessary and are therefore incorrect.

14. The nurse is guiding a mother through the treatment for enterobiasis. Which instruction should be included in the teaching plan?

a. Intravenous antibiotic therapy will be ordered.

b. Medication therapy will continue for one year.

c. The entire family should be treated.

d. Treatment is not recommended for children under the age of 10 years.

Answer C is correct. Pinworms (enterobiasis) is treated using Vermox (mebendazole) or Antiminth (pyrantel pamoate). To make sure no worms remain, it is important that the entire family is treated. The family should get tested again after two weeks. Answers A, B and D do not apply and are therefore incorrect.

15. Lidocaine is a medication frequently prescribed for the client experiencing:

a. Atrial tachycardia

b. Heart block

c. Ventricular brachycardia

d. Ventricular tachycardia

Answer D is correct. Lidocaine increases the electric stimulation threshold of the ventricles without depressing the force of ventricular contractions, thereby exerting an antiarrhythmic effect. The medication is therefore used in the treatment of ventricular tachycardia. Answer A is incorrect because Lidocaine is not used for atrial arrhythmias. Answers B and C are incorrect because Lidocaine slows down the heart rate and it is therefore not used for brachycardia or heart block.

16. The client is scheduled for a Tensilon test to check for Myasthenia Gravis. Which of the following drugs should be kept available during the test?

a. Atropine sulfate

b. Promethazine

c. Prostigmin

d. Furosemide

Answer A is correct. This is because atropine sulfate is the antidote for Tensilon and is therefore used to treat cholenergic crises. Answers B, C, and D are all incorrect. Answer B is incorrect because Promethazine is an antiemetic anti-anxiety medication. Answer C is incorrect because Prostigmin is utilized to treat myasthenia gravis. Answer D is incorrect as Furosemide is a diuretic.

17. Which of the following should be used in the treatment of iron toxicity?

a. Desferal (deferoxamine)

b. Digibind (digoxin immune Fab)

c. Narcan (naloxone)

d. Zinecard (dexrazoxane)

Answer A is correct. Desferal is used to treat iron toxicity. Answer B is incorrect because Digibind is used to treat dioxin toxicity. Answer C is incorrect because Narcan is used to treat narcotic overdose. Answer D is incorrect because is utilized to treat doxorubicin toxicity. Answers B, C, and D are all antidotes for other medications.

18. The physician has prescribed Amoxil (amoxicillin) 500mg capsules for a client with esophageal varices. The nurse can best care for the client by:

a. Administering the medication with an antacid

b. Giving the client the medication as ordered

c. Providing extra water with the medication

d. Requesting the medication in an alternative form an alternate form of the medication

Answer D is correct. The client with esophageal varices could potentially develop spontaneous bleeding from the mechanical irritation caused by taking capsules. Because of this, the nurse should request an alternate form of the medication, for example a suspension. Answer A is incorrect because Amoxil should not be given with milk or antacids. Answer B is incorrect because this would not be in the best interest of the client. Answer C is incorrect because providing extra water is not a good means of preventing bleeding.

19. The physician has prescribed Dilantin (phenytoin) 100mg for a client with generalized tonic clonic seizures to be administered intravenously. The nurse should administer the medication:

a. Rapidly with an IV push

b. Through a small vein

c. With IV dextrose

d. Slowly over 2–3 minutes

Answer D is correct. Dilantin should be administered slowly – no more than 50mg per minute as cardiac arrhythmias can otherwise occur. Answer A is incorrect because the drug must be administered slowly. Answers B and C are also incorrect. Dextrose solutions cause the medication to crystallize in the line and the medication should therefore be administered through a large vein in order to prevent "purple glove" syndrome.

20. The nurse finds that the respiratory rate of a post-operative client has dropped from 14 breaths per minute to 6 breaths per minute. The nurse gives the client Narcan (naloxone) as per standing order. After Narcan has been administered, the nurse should assess the client for:

a. Projectile vomiting

b. Pupillary changes

c. Sudden, intense pain

d. Wheezing respirations

Answer C is correct. The medication Narcan is a narcotic antagonist that blocks the effects of the client's pain medication. Because of this, the client will experience sudden, intense pain. Answers A, B, and D are incorrect because they do not relate to the condition of the client in relation to the administration of Narcan.

21. A client with congestive heart failure has been maintained with digoxin (Lanoxin). Which of the following indicates that the drug is having a desired effect?

a. Improved appetite

b. Increased pedal edema

c. Increased urinary output

d. Stabilized weight

Answer C is correct. The medication slows and strengthens the contraction of the heart. An increase in urinary output therefore shows that Lanoxin is having a desired effect by eliminating excess fluid from the body. Answers A, B, and D are all incorrect. Answer A is incorrect because it is not related to the medication. Answer B is incorrect because pedal edema would decrease and not increase. Answer D is incorrect because the client's weight would decrease.

22. The physician has prescribed the medication Basaljel (aluminum carbonate gel) for a client with recurrent indigestion. The nurse should inform the client of the side effects that come from using the medication, which include:

a. Confusion

b. Constipation

c. Diarrhea

d. Urinary retention

Answer B is correct. Constipation is a common side effect of Basaljel, which is an antacid that contains aluminum. Answers A, C, and D are all incorrect as they are not common side effects of the medication.

23. A client in labor has an order for Demerol (meperidine) 75 mg. IM which is to be administered 10 minutes before delivery. The nurse should:

a. Administer the medication as ordered

b. Administer the medication IM during the delivery to prevent pain from the episiotomy

c. Question the order

d. Wait until the client is placed on the delivery table then give the medication

Answer C is correct. Giving a narcotic to a pregnant client close to the time of delivery can result in respiratory depression in the newborn. Because of this, the nurse should question the order. Answers A, B, and D are all incorrect for the very same reason.

24. The physician has ordered Synthroid (levothyroxine) for a client with myxedema. Which statement shows that the client understands the nurse's instruction regarding the medication?

a. "I will check my heart rate before taking the medication."

b. "I will take the medication every morning after breakfast."

c. "If I develop gastric upset, I will stop taking the medication."

d. "If I experience any visual disturbance, I will report this to my doctor."

Answer A is correct. The client should be instructed and taught to the check their heart rate before taking the medication. This is because Synthroid (levothyroxine) increases metabolic rate and cardiac output and adverse reactions to the medication include tachycardia and dysrhythmias. Answer B is incorrect because the client does not have to take the medication after breakfast. Answer C is incorrect as the medication should not be stopped if the client develops gastric upset. Answer D is also incorrect because it has no relation to the medication.

25. A client who has recently been diagnosed with diabetes has started receiving Precose (acarbose). The nurse should instruct the client to take the medication:

a. 1 hour before meals

b. 30 minutes after meals

c. Every day at bedtime

d. With the first bite of a meal

Answer D is correct. The medication should be taken with the first bite of a meal. Answers A, B and C are all incorrect.

26. A 6-year-old client is being treated for an acute attack of asthma using racemic epinephrine (epinephrine hydrochloride) nebulizer stat. Which of the following indicates an adverse effect of this medication?

a. Excitability
b. Heart rate 150
c. Nausea
d. Tremors

Answer B is correct. This is because hypertension and tachycardia are both adverse effects of epinephrine. Answers A, C, and D are all incorrect in this case as these are expected side effects of racemic epinephrine.

27. The client is being treated with intravenous Vancomycin for MRSA. The nurse notices redness of the neck and chest of the client. Place in ordered sequence the actions that the nurse should take:

a. Administer Benadryl as ordered
b. Call the doctor
c. Stop the IV infusion of Vancomycin
d. Take the vital signs

The correct order is C, D, B, A.

28. A client with leukemia has been receiving oral prednisolone (Prednisone). Which of the following is an expected side effect of the prolonged use of prednisolone?

a. Decreased appetite
b. Hirsutism
c. Integumentary bronzing
d. Weight loss

Answer B is correct. Hirsutism, or facial hair, is a side effect of cortisone therapy. Answers A, C, and D are all incorrect. These are symptoms of Addison's disease.

29. The physician has prescribed DDAVP (desmopressin acetate) for a client with diabetes insipidus. Which of the following is an indication that the medication is having a desired effect?

a. A decline in the client's urinary output
b. An increase in the client's activity level
c. The client has an improved appetite
d. The client's morning blood sugar was 120mg/dL

Answer A is correct. A declined in urinary output shows that the drug is having its desired effects. This is because excessive production of dilute urine is a characteristic of diabetes insipidus. Answers B and C are incorrect as they are not related to the question. Answer D is incorrect as it refers to diabetes mellitus.

30. A 15-year-old client with cystic acne has an order for Accutane (isotretinoin). Prior to starting the medication, which lab work is needed?

a. Clean-catch urinalysis

b. Liver profile

c. Complete blood count

d. Thyroid function test

Answer B is correct. The medication Accutane consists of concentrated vitamin A, which is a fat-soluble vitamin. A liver panel is needed as fat-soluble vitamins can potentially become hepatotoxic. Answers A, C, and D are incorrect as they do not relate to therapy with Accutane.

31. A post-operative client has a prescription for Demerol (meperidine) 75mg and Phenergan (promethazine) 25mg IM every 3–4 hours as required to counter pain. When taken in combination, the two medications produce:

a. A Excitatory effect

b. A Synergistic effect

c. An Agonist effect

d. An Antagonist effect

Answer B is correct. The two medications when taken in combination produce a synergistic effect, that is, an effect that is greater than that of either drug used alone. Answer A is incorrect because the two drugs combined would have a depressing effect, and not an excitatory effect. Answer C is incorrect because agonist effects are similar to those produced by chemicals normally present in the body. Answer D is incorrect because antagonist effects are those in which the actions of the medications oppose one another.

32. Prior to giving a client's morning dose of Lanoxin (digoxin), the nurse checks the apical pulse rate. She finds a rate of 54. The appropriate nursing intervention in this instance is to:

a. Administer the medication and monitor the heart rate

b. Record the pulse rate and administer the medication

c. Withhold the medication and notify the doctor

d. Withhold the medication until the heart rate increases

Answer C is correct. The appropriate nursing intervention in this scenario is to best provide for the client's safety by withholding the medication and notify the doctor. Answers A, B, and D are incorrect.

33. A client with schizophrenia has started receiving Zyprexa (olanzapine). Three weeks later, the client

develops severe muscle rigidity and elevated temperature. The nurse should give priority to which of the following interventions:

a. Administering prescribed anti-Parkinsonian medication

b. Ordering a CBC and CPK

c. Transferring the client to a medical unit

d. Withholding all morning medications

Answer A is correct. Severe muscle rigidity and elevated temperature are symptoms that suggest that the client is experiencing an adverse reaction to the medication known as as neuroleptic malignant syndrome. Answers B, C, and D are incorrect as they are not appropriate interventions.

34. A child with cystic fibrosis is receiving inhalation therapy with Pulmozyme (dornase alfa). Which of the following is a side effect of the medication?

a. Brittle nails

b. Hair loss

c. Sore throat

d. Weight gain

Answer C is correct. Side effects of Pulmozyme include hoarseness, laryngitis, sore throat. Answers A, B, and D are incorrect because they are not associated with Pulmozyme.

35. A client who has been maintained with Dilantin (phenytoin) for tonic-clonic seizures is preparing for discharge. Which of the following should be included in the client's discharge care plan?

a. A high-carbohydrate diet must be avoided

b. Regularly scheduled blood work will be needed

c. The medication can cause dental staining

d. The medication can cause problems with drowsiness

Answer B is correct. The client will need regularly scheduled blood work because agranulocytosis and aplastic anemia are potential adverse side effects of Dilantin. Answer A is incorrect because the drug does not interfere with the metabolism of carbohydrates. Answer C is incorrect because Dilantin does not cause dental staining. Answer D is incorrect because Dilantn does not cause any problems related to drowsiness.

36. The doctor has prescribed Cortone (cortisone) for a client with systemic lupus erythematosis. Which instruction should be given to the client?

a. Report changes in appetite and weight to the doctor

b. Schedule a time to take the influenza vaccine every year

c. Take the medication 30 minutes before meals

d. Wear sunglasses to prevent cataracts

Answer B is correct. This is because a client who is receiving steroid medication should also receive an annual influenza vaccine. Answer A is incorrect because weight gain and an increased appetite are both expected side effects of steroid medication. Answer C is incorrect because the medication should be taken with meals. Answer D is incorrect because wearing sunglasses does not prevent cataracts in the client taking Cortone.

37. The physician has prescribed Stadol (butorphanol) for a post-operative client. The nurse knows that the medication is having its desired effect if the client:

a. Has an increased urinary output

b. Is asleep for 30 minutes after the injection

c. Reports that he/she is feeling less nauseated

d. States that he/she is still feeling hungry

Answer B is correct. The medication reduces the perception of pain, which allows the post-operative client to rest. Answers A and D are incorrect as these are not affected by the medication. Answer C is incorrect because, although pain relief can reduce symptoms of nausea, it is not a desired effect of the Stadol.

38. A client is hospitalized with hepatitis A. Which of the client's regular medications is contraindicated due to the current illness?

a. Lipitor (atorvastatin)

b. Premarin (conjugated estrogens)

c. Prilosec (omeprazole)

d. Synthroid (levothyroxine)

Answer A is correct. Lipid-lowering agents are contraindicated in the client with active liver disease. Answers B, C, and D are incorrect as they are not contraindicated in the client with active liver disease.

39. A client with diabetes mellitus has a prescription for Glucotrol XL (glipizide). The client should be instructed to take the medication:

a. With breakfast

b. Before lunch

c. After dinner

d. At bedtime

Answer A is correct. Glucotrol XL is to be taken once a day with breakfast. Answers B and C are incorrect because the client would hypoglycemia later in the day or evening. Answer D is incorrect because the client would also develop hypoglycemia while sleeping.

40. The physician has prescribed Vancocin (vancomycin) 500mg IV every six hours for a client with MRSA. The medication should be administered in the following manner:

a. IV push

b. Over 15 minutes

c. Over 30 minutes

d. Over 60 minutes

Answer D is correct. The medication should be given very slowly so as to prevent "redman" syndrome. Answer A is incorrect because Vancomycin is not given IV push. Answers B and C are also incorrect because the medication should be administered at a slower rate.

41. The nurse calculates the amount of an antibiotic for injection to be administered to an infant. The amount of medication to be given is 1.25mL. Which of the following is the correct way to administer the antibiotic?

a. Administer the medication in one injection in the dorsogluteal muscle

b. Administer the medication in one injection in the ventrogluteal muscle

c. Divide the amount in two injections and administer one in the ventrogluteal muscle and one in the vastus lateralis muscle

d. Divide the amount into two injections and administer in each vastus lateralis muscle

Answer D is correct. This is because no more than 1mL should be administered in the vastus lateralis of an infant. Answers A, B, and C are all incorrect because the other two muscles, the dorsogluteal and ventrogluteal muscles, are not used for injections in the infant.

42. An 65-year-old client with glaucoma is scheduled for a cholecystectomy. Which of the following drug prescriptions should the nurse question?

a. Atropine (atropine)
b. Demerol (meperidine)
c. Phenergan (promethazine)
d. Tagamet (cimetadine)

Answer A is correct. This is because Atropine increases intraocular pressure and is contraindicated in the client with glaucoma. Answers B, C, and D are incorrect as they are not contraindicated in the client with glaucoma.

43. The physician has prescribed Dilantin (phenytoin) for a client with generalized seizures. When planning the client's care, the nurse should:

a. Check the client's pulse prior to administering the medication

b. Give the medication 30 minutes before meals

c. Maintain strict intake and output

d. Provide oral hygiene and gum care at every shift

Answer D is correct. The nurse should provide oral hygiene and gum care at every shift because Gingival hyperplasia is a side effect of Dilantin. Answers A, B, and C are incorrect because they do not apply to the medication.

44. The physician has ordered Cognex (tacrine) for a client with dementia. The nurse should monitor the client for potential adverse reactions, which include:

a. Hypoglycemia

b. Jaundice

c. Tinnitus

d. Urinary retention

Answer B is correct. The nurse should monitor the client for any symptoms of jaundice. This is because drug-induced hepatitis is an adverse reaction associated to Cognex. Answers A, C, and D are incorrect because these are not among the adverse reactions that can be linked to the medication.

45. A client exhibiting serum cholesterol of 275mg/dL is placed on rosuvastatin (Crestor). Which instruction should a nurse give to a client using rosuvastatin (Crestor)?

a. Allow 6 months for the drug to take effect
b. Report any signs of insomnia
c. Report any signs of muscle weakness to the doctor
d. Take the medication with fruit juice

Answer C is correct. Crestor is an antilipidemic drug. A client using Crestor must therefore report any signs of muscle weakness as these may be symptomatic of rhabdomyolysis. Answer A is incorrect because the drug takes effect in the first month of starting therapy. Answer B is incorrect because it is unrelated to Crestor. Answer D is also incorrect because mixing the medication with fruit juice, particularly grapefruit, can decrease its effectiveness. Crestor should always be taken with water.

46. The physician prescribes lisinopril (Zestril) and furosemide (Lasix) to be administered concomitantly to the client with hypertension. The appropriate nursing intervention is to:

a. Administer both medications

b. Administer the medications separately

c. Contact the pharmacy

d. Question the order

Answer A is correct. Zestril is an ACE inhibitor and Lasix is a diuretic for hypertension. ACE inhibitors are frequently given with diuretics and the nurse should therefore administer both medications. Answers B, C, and D are all incorrect. There is no need to administer the medications separately, to question the order, or contact the pharmacy.

47. The client with varicella will most likely have a prescription for which category of medication?

a. Antibiotics

b. Anticoagulants

c. Antipyretics

d. Antivirals

Answer D is correct. Varicella (chicken pox) is a herpes virus which is best treated with antiviral medications. Answer A and B are both incorrect because the client is not treated with antibiotics or anticoagulants. Answer C is also incorrect because even though the client may have a fever before the chicken pox appear, the temperature will usually go down.

48. A client with urinary tract infection has a prescription for Pyridium (phenazopyridine hydrochloride). The nurse should inform that client that the medication may:

a. Cause changes in taste

b. Cause diarrhea

c. Cause mental confusion

d. Turn her urine orange or red

Answer D is correct. A nurse should teach clients taking Pyridium that the medication will change the color of her urine. The medication, if taken in large doses, can also result in sclera and pale or yellowed skin. Answers A, B, and C are incorrect as diarrhea, mental confusion or changes in taste are not side effects of the medication.

49. A client who has recently undergone a heart transplant is started on medication to prevent organ rejection. Which of the below drug categories prevent the formation of antibodies against the new organ?

a. Analgesics

b. Antibiotics

c. Antivirals

d. Immunosuppressants

Answer D is correct. Immunosuppressants are utilized to prevent the formation of antibodies. Answers A, B, and C are incorrect because analgesics, antibiotics, and antivirals are not used to prevent antibody production.

50. A physician has ordered streptokinase for a client. Before administering the medication, the nurse should check the client for:

a. A history of alcohol abuse

b. A history of streptococcal infections

c. Allergies to pineapples and bananas

d. Prior therapy with phenytoin

Answer B is correct. This is because clients with a history of streptococcal infections could have antibodies that make streptokinase ineffective. Answers A, C, and D are incorrect. There is no reason to assess the client for a history of alcohol abuse, allergies to pineapples or bananas, and there is also no correlation to the use of phenytoin and streptokinase.

51. The nurse has received a pre-op order to administer Valium (diazepam) 10mg and Phenergan (promethazine) 25mg. The correct process of administering these medications is to:

a. Question the order because they the two medications cannot be given at the same time

b. Administer the Valium first and to wait five minutes before injecting the Phenergan

c. Administer the medications separately

d. Administer both medications together in one syringe

Answer C is correct. Valium is an anti-anxiety drug and Phenergan is an antiemetic. The medications should be administered separately but can be given to the client at the same time. Answer A is incorrect because the two medications can be given to the same client. Answer B is incorrect as there is no need to wait to inject the second medication. Answer D is incorrect because Valium should not be given in same syringe with other medications.

52. The physician has ordered Cobex (cyanocobalamin) for a client following a gastric resection. Which finding indicates that the medication is having its intended effect?

a. Platelet count of 250,000 cu. mm

b. Neutrophil count of 4500 cu mm

c. Hgb of 14.2 g/dL

d. Eeosinophil count of 200 cu mm

Answer C is correct. The medication Cobex is an injectable form of vitamin B12 or cyanocobalamin. A lab finding showing an increase in Hgb levels shows that the medication is effective. Answers A, B, and D are incorrect as they are not indicative of the effectiveness of the medication.

53. A client with paranoid schizophrenia has a prescription for Thorazine (chlorpromazine) 400mg orally twice daily. Which of the following symptoms should immediately be reported to the physician?

a. Lethargy, slurred speech, thirst
b. Fever, sore throat, weakness
c. Fatigue, drowsiness, photosensitivity
d. Dry mouth, constipation, blurred vision

Answer B is correct. Any symptoms of fever, sore throat, and weakness should be reported immediately. Agranulocytosis is a potential adverse effect of Thorazine, which renders the client vulnerable to overwhelming infection. Answers A, C, and D are expected side effects and there is therefore no need to notify the physician immediately.

54. The doctor has prescribed an infusion of Osmitrol (mannitol) for a client with increased intracranial pressure. Which of the following findings indicates the direct effectiveness of the drug?

a. An increased urinary output

b. An increased pupil size

c. An increased pulse rate

d. A decreased diastolic blood pressure

Answer A is correct. Osmitrol (mannitol) is an osmotic diuretic, which inhibits reabsorption of sodium and water. An increased urinary output is therefore a direct indication of the effectiveness of the drug. Answers B, C, and D are incorrect as they do not relate to the effectiveness of the drug.

55. The client with a urinary tract infection has an order for Gantrisin (sulfasoxazole) 1gm in divided doses. The nurse should administer the medication:

a. With meals or a snack
b. 30 minutes before meals
c. 30 minutes after meals
d. At bedtime

Answer B is correct. To enhance absorption, Sulfa drugs, including Gantrisin, should be administered 30 minutes before meals. Answer A is incorrect because the drug should be administered prior to meals. Answer C is incorrect because the medication should always be given on an empty stomach. Answer D is incorrect as the medication should be administered in divided doses throughout the course of the day.

56. The mother of a child with chickenpox is inquiring whether there is a medication that can help reduce the course of chickenpox. Which of the following medications can be used to speed up healing of the lesions and thereby shorten the duration of fever and itching?

a. Periactin (cyproheptadine)

b. Varivax (varicella vaccine)

c. VZIG (varicella-zoster immune globulin)

d. Zovirax (acyclovir)

Answer D is correct. Zovirax shortens the course of chickenpox, but the American Academy of Pediatrics does not recommend it for healthy children because of the cost. Answer A is incorrect because Periactin is an antihistamine that is used to control itching that results from chickenpox. Answer B is incorrect because Varivax is the vaccine that is used to prevent chickenpox. Answer C is also incorrect as VZIG is the immune globulin that is given to those who have become exposed to chicken pox.

57. The physician has ordered Chloromycetin (chloramphenicol) for a client with bacterial meningitis. The nurse should pay particular attention to the following lab report:

a. Complete blood count

b. Serum creatinine

c. Serum sodium

d. Urine specific gravity

Answer A is correct. The nurse should monitor the client's complete blood count most carefully. This is because aplastic anemia is an adverse side effect of chloramphenico. Answers B, C, and D are not directly affected by the medication and are therefore incorrect. Nevertheless, these should be noted down by the nurse.

58. A client admitted for treatment of bacterial pneumonia has a prescription for intravenous ampicillin. Which specimen should the nurse obtain before administering the medication?

a. Complete blood count

b. Routine urinalysis

c. Serum electrolytes

d. Sputum for culture and sensitivity

Answer D is correct. The nurse should obtain a sputum specimen for culture and sensitivity before administering the antibiotic in order to check whether the organism is sensitive to the prescribed medication. A, B, and C are all incorrect as a routine urinalysis, complete blood count, and serum electrolytes can be obtained after the therapy has commenced.

59. The client with angina has an order for nitroglycerin sublingual tablets. The nurse should instruct the client to take the medication:

a. After engaging in light exercise

b. As soon as the client notices signs of chest pain

c. At bedtime to prevent nocturnal angina

d. Every four hours to prevent chest pain

Answer B is correct. The client should take the medication as soon as he notices chest pain or discomfort. Answer A is incorrect because the tablets should be taken before engaging in activity. Any strenuous activity should be avoided. Answer C is incorrect because the drugs do not prevent nocturnal angina. Answer D is incorrect because the tablets should be taken when the pain occurs and not according to a regular schedule.

60. The client is maintained on Lugol's solution prior to a thyroidectomy. The nurse should instruct the client to:

a. Take the solution at bedtime

b. Take the medication with juice

c. Report changes in appetite

d. Avoid sunshine while taking the medication

Answer B is correct. Lugol's solution is a soluble solution of potassium iodine and because of its bitter taste, it should be given with juice. Answer A is incorrect. Answer C and D are both unnecessary and therefore also incorrect.

61. A client is to receive Dilantin (phenytoin) via a nasogastric (NG) tube. When administering the drug, the nurse should:

a. Administer the medication, flush with 5mL of water, and clamp the NG tube

b. Flush the NG tube with 2–4mL of water before administering the medication

c. Flush the NG tube with 2–4oz of water before and after giving the medication

d. Flush the NG tube with 5mL of normal saline and give the medication

Answer C is correct. When administering the medication, the nurse should flush the NG tube twice with 2–4oz of water, that is, before and after giving the medication. Answers A and B are incorrect because insufficient amounts of water are used in both options. Answer D is incorrect because saline should not be used to flush the NG tube.

62. A client with pneumocystis carinii has an order for Pentam (pentamidine) IV. While receiving the medication, the nurse should carefully monitor the client's:

a. Blood pressure

b. Heart rate

c. Respirations

d. Temperature

Answer A is correct. This is because hypotension is a severe toxic side effect of pentamidine. Answers B, C, and D are incorrect as they are unrelated.

63. A client in labor has received epidural anesthesia with Marcaine (bupivacaine). Epidural anesthesia produces vasodilation which results in a decrease in blood pressure. To reverse the hypotension caused by epidural anesthesia, the nurse should have which medication nearby?

a. Adrenalin (epinephrine)

b. Dobutrex (dobutamine)

c. Narcan (naloxone)

d. Romazicon (flumazenil)

Answer A is correct. The nurse should make sure to have adrenalin available to reverse hypotension. Answer B is incorrect because Dobutrex is an adrenergic which increases cardiac output. Answer C is incorrect because Nracan is a narcotic antagonist. Answer D is likewise incorrect because Romazicon is a benzodiazepine antagonist.

64. Four clients are to receive medication. Which client should the nurse prioritise?

a. The client with abdominal surgery receiving Phenergan (promethazine) IM every four hours PRN for nausea and vomiting

b. The client with an apical pulse of 72 receiving Lanoxin (digoxin) PO daily

c. The client with labored respirations receiving a stat dose of IV Lasix (furosemide)

d. The client with pneumonia receiving Polycillin (ampicillin) IVPB every six hours

Answer C is correct. The client receiving a stat dose of IV Lasix should be first to receive his medication. Answers A, B, and D are incorrect because these are regularly scheduled medications for clients whose conditions are more stable.

65. The physician has ordered an injection of morphine for a client with post-operative pain. Before giving the medication, the nurse should check the client's:

a. Blood pressure

b. Heart rate

c. Respirations

d. Temperature

Answer C is correct. It is absolutely essential for the nurse to assess the client's respirations. This is because Morphine is an opiate and can therefore severely depress the client's respirations. Answers A, B, and D are incorrect.

66. A client with AIDS tells the nurse that she regularly takes echinacea to boost her immune system. The nurse should inform the client that:

a. Herbals can interfere with the action of antiviral medication

b. Herbals have been shown to decrease the viral load

c. Supplements appear to prevent replication of the virus

d. Supplements have proven effective in prolonging life

Answer A is correct. The nurse should advise the client to discuss the use of herbals with his doctor because herbal remedies such as echinacea can interfere with the action of antiviral medications. Answer B is incorrect as it has not been shown that herbals can reduce the viral load. Answer C is incorrect because herbals do not prevent replication of the virus. Answer D is incorrect because it has not been shown that herbals can prolong life.

67. The physician has ordered Activase (alteplase) for a client admitted with a myocardial infarction. Which of the following is a desired effect of Activase?

a. An increased tissue oxygenation

b. The destruction of the clot

c. The prevention of congestive heart failure

d. The stabilization of the clot

Answer B is correct. The desired effect of Activase, a thrombolytic agent, is to destroy the clot. Answer A is incorrect because increased oxygenation is not a direct result of the medication. Answer C is incorrect because Axtivase does not prevent congestive heart failure. Answer D is incorrect because the medication does not stabilize the clot.

68. A client informs the nurse that she takes St. John's wort (hypericum perforatum) three times a day to counter mild depression. The nurse should advise the client that:

a. It is safe to use the herbal with other antidepressants

b. She should avoid eating aged cheese

c. Skin reactions increase with the use of sunscreen

d. The herbal St. John's wort seldom rarely depression

Answer B is correct. The herbal St. John's wort has properties similar to those of monoamine oxidase inhibitors (MAOI). Therefore, eating foods high in tryramine such as aged cheese, chocolate, salami, and liver can result in a hypertensive crisis. Answer A is incorrect because the herbal should not be used in combination with MAOI antidepressants. Answer C is incorrect because use of a sunscreen prevents skin reactions to sun exposure. Answer D is likewise incorrect because St. John's wort can relieve mild to moderate depression.

69. A client with chronic pain is being treated with opioid administration via epidural route. Which medication should be kept nearby and available due to a possible complication of this pain relief procedure?

a. Diphenhydramine (Benadryl)

b. Ketorolac (Toradol)

c. Naloxone (Narcan)

d. Promethazine (Phenergan)

Answer C is correct. Naloxene should be kept nearby as an antagonist for these medications. This is because Rrspiratory depression can occur from the administration of opioids. Answers A, B, and D are not necessarily incorrect as they might also be needed, but respiratory depression is the most important and most sever problem that could occur. Benadryl and Phenergan may however be used to treat itching and nausea. Toradol, which is classified as an NSAID, could be used for its anti-inflammatory properties.

70. The nurse is checking the medication history of a client who was admitted for surgery in the morning. Which long-term medication in the client's history would be most important to report to the doctor?

a. Docusate (Colace)

b. Lisinopril (Zestril)

c. Oscal D

d. Prednisone

Answer D is correct. The nurse should definitely report usage of prednisone. This is because a sudden withdrawal of steroids could potentially lead to a collapse of the cardiovascular system. Answer A, B, and C are incorrect as these are not so relevant in the maintenance of the steroids. Colace is a stool softener, Zestril is an ACE inhibitor used as an antihypertensive, and Oscal D is a calcium and vitamin agent.

71. A nurse is working in an endoscopy recovery area. To provide conscious sedation, many of the clients are given midazolam (Versed). Which drug should always be available as an antidote for Versed?

a. Diazepam (Valium)

b. Florinef (Fludrocortisone)

c. Flumazenil (Romazicon)

d. Naloxone (Narcan)

Answer C is correct. Romazicon, a benzodiazepine, is the antidote for Versed, which is used as an antianxiety drug and for conscious sedation. Answers A, B, and D are incorrect as these medications are not used antagonists for Versed.

72. A client with asthma has a prescription to start an aminophylline IV infusion. Which of the following is essential for the nurse to safely administer the medication?

a. Cover to prevent exposure of solution to light

b. IV infusion device

c. IV inline filter

d. Large bore intravenous catheter

Answer B is correct. An infusion device should be used to regulate Aminophylline, thereby preventing improper infusion rates. Answers A, C, and D are incorrect as they are not necessary for administration of this medication.

73. A client with osteoporosis is being discharged on alendronate (Fosamax). Which statement would indicate a need for further teaching?

a. "After taking Fosamax, I should remain in an upright position for 30 minutes."

b. "I should not have any food with this medication."

c. "I should take Fosamax orally with water."

d. "I should take the medication immediately every night before bedtime."

Answer D is correct. Fosamax should be taken in the morning before taking any other medications and before having food. The medication should be taken with water as the only liquid. Statement D is therefore incorrect and is a sign that further teaching is required. All other answers (A, B, and C) are correct administrations.

74. A client has an order for Demerol 75mg and atropine 0.4mg IM as a preoperative medication. The Demerol vial contains 50mg/mL, and atropine is available 0.4mg/mL. The nurse should administer how much medication in total?

a. 1.0mL

b. 1.7mLs

c. 2.5mLs

d. 3.0 mLs

Answer C is correct. The calculated dosage of Atropine is 1.0mL, and the calculated dosage of Demerol is 1.5mL, which comes to a total of 2.5mL. Answers A, B, and D are all incorrect calculations.

75. The nurse is discharging a client with asthma with a prescription for zafirlukast (Accolate). Which statement by the client would indicate a need for further teaching?

a. "I should take this medication when eating."

b. "If I'm already having an asthma attack, this drug will not stop it."

c. "My doctor might order liver tests while I'm on this drug."

d. "Should I experience any flu-like symptoms, I should report this to my doctor."

Answer A is correct. the medication should be taken either one hour before or two hours after meals. This is to prevent slow absorption of the drug. Statement A is therefore incorrect and is a sign that further teaching is required. Answers B, C, and D are all correct statements.

76. A physician has prescribed haloperidol (Haldol) for a client with advanced Alzheimer's disease. Which of the following symptoms suggests that the client is experiencing side effects from this drug?

a. Cough

b. Diarrhea

c. Pitting edema

d. Tremors

Answer D is correct. When taking Haldol, tremors are an extrapyramidal side effect that can occur. Answers A, B, and C are all incorrect and are not side or adverse effects of the medication.

77. A client with Alzheimer's disease has an order for donepezil (Aricept). Which information should the nurse always include in the teaching plan for a client who is placed on Aricept?

a. "If a dose is skipped, take two the next time."

b. "Rise slowly because the medicine can cause dizziness."

c. "Take the medication with meals."

d. "The pill can cause your heart rate to increase."

Answer B is correct. Dizziness is a side effect of Aricept and the client should therefore be advised to move slowly when rising from a sitting or lying position. Answer A is incorrect because increasing the number of pills the client takes can increase the side effects and is therefore not recommended. Answer C is incorrect because the medication should be taken at bedtime, with no regard to food. Answer D is also incorrect because bradycardia is another effect of the medication.

78. The client has a cocaine addiction. The nurse should expect the client to be placed on which medication?

a. Bromocriptine (Parlodel)

b. Disulfiram (Antabuse)

c. Methadone

d. THC

Answer A is correct. Bromocriptine (Parlodel) is classified as an anti-Parkinsonism drug and gives clients with this addiction a substitute for the neurotransmitter dopamine. It is therefore the medication utilized for addiction to cocaine. Answer B is incorrect because Antabuse is used for alcohol abuse. Answer C is incorrect as Methadone is used for opioid addiction. Answer D is also incorrect as THC is marijuana and is not utilized for replacement therapy.

79. A client has been placed on the drug valproic acid (Depakene). Which of the following symptoms would indicate to the nurse that the client is experiencing an adverse reaction to the drug?

a. Lethargy

b. Photophobia

c. Poor skin turgor

d. Reported visual disturbances

Answer A is correct. This is because Lethargy could be an indication of hepatatoxicity. The nurse should carefully monitor for any signs of anorexia, nausea, jaundice, facial edema, vomiting, and unusual bleeding or bruising. Answers B, C, and D are incorrect as they are not clinical manifestations of adverse effects of the drug Depakene.

80. A client with a diagnosis of Amyotrophic Lateral Sclerosis (ALS) has received a prescription riluzole (Rilutek). Which instructions should the nurse include when teaching the client about this medication? Select all that apply.

a. Avoid any use of alcohol

b. Laboratory test will be monitored regularly

c. Medication should be taken at the same time each day

d. Report any fever to the health care provider

e. Take the medication with meals

Answers A, B, C, and D are all correct. A client placed on Rilutek should avoid using alcohol, report any signs of fever, and take the medication at the same time each day. These factors, along with the monitoring of laboratory values are all information that should be included in the teaching plan. Answer E is incorrect because the medication should not be taken with food.

81. The nurse is caring for a client with leukemia who has been maintained with doxorubicin (Adriamycin). Which toxic effects of this medication should the nurse immediately report to the physician?

a. Elevated BUN and dry, flaky skin

b. Nausea and vomiting

c. Rales and distended neck veins

d. Red discoloration of the urine

Answer C is correct. The medication can cause cardiotoxicity exhibited by changes in the ECG and congestive heart failure. Rales and distended neck veins are clinical manifestations of congestive heart failure and must be reported immediately. Answer A is incorrect as this effect is not specific to the medication. Answer B is incorrect because nausea and vomiting is a common side effect and therefore there is no need to report this immediately to the doctor. Answer D is incorrect because the reddish discoloration of the urine is a harmless side effect of the medication.

82. The nurse is performing an admission history for a client recovering from a stroke. The client's dedication history reveals that the client has been taking clopidogrel (Plavix). Which clinical manifestation alerts the nurse to an adverse effect of this medication?

a. Epistaxis

b. Hyperactivity

c. Hypothermia

d. Nausea

Answer A is correct. The medication Plavix is an antiplatelet and therefore epistaxis, bleeding from the nose, could indicate a severe effect. Answers B, C, and D have no direct relation to the undesired effects of the medication.

83. A client with angina is experiencing migraines and has received a prescription for Sumatriptan succinate (Imitrex). Which of the following nursing actions is most appropriate?

a. Call the doctor to question the prescription order

b. Consult social services for financial assistance with obtaining the drug

c. Perform discharge teaching for this medication

d. Try to obtain samples for the client to take home

Answer A is correct. Answer A is most appropriate in this scenario. The medication results in

cranial vasoconstriction to reduce pain, but can also cause vasoconstrictive effects. Because of this, it is contraindicated in clients who have angina. Therefore, it is necessary to contact and notify the doctor. Answer C is appropriate also, but answer A is more appropriate. Answers B and D are incorrect. These are both inappropriate actions.

84. A client with increased intracranial pressure is maintained on Furosemide (Lasix) and Osmitrol (Mannitol). The nurse recognizes that these two medications are administered to reverse which effect?

a. Cellular edema

b. Energy failure

c. Excessive glutamate release

d. Excessive intracellular calcium

Answer A is correct. The medications Lasix and Mannitol are given for their diuretic effects in decreasing cerebral edema. Answers C, B, and D are therefore incorrect.

85. A client has an order for cisplatin (Platinol). Which medication would the nurse expect to be ordered in order to reduce renal toxicity from the cisplatin infusion?

a. Pamidronate (Aredia)

b. Mesna (Mesenex)

c. Dexrazoxane (Zinecard)

d. Amifostine (Ethyol)

Answer D is correct. The drug Ethyol is used to reduce renal toxicity with cisplatin administration. Answers A, B, and C are therefore incorrect as these drugs are cytoprotectants which are not utilized for cisplatin administration.

86. A client with a ruptured cerebral aneurysm has received an order for Nimodipine (Nimotop). Which of the following is a desired effect of this drug?

a. Restoration of a normal blood pressure reading

b. Prevention of the influx of calcium into cells

c. Prevention of the inflammatory process

d. Dissolving of the clot that has formed

Answer B is correct. The medication Nimotop is a calcium channel blocker that is used to prevent calcium influx. The causation of vasospasm of the blood vessel is thought to be related to this calcium influx. Because of this, Nimotop is administered to prevent this. Answers A, C, and D are incorrect as they do not describe the action of this drug.

87. The client with erosive gastritis has been placed on Nexium (esomeprazole). The nurse should administer the drug:

a. With each meal

b. In a single dose at bedtime

c. 30 minutes before a meal

d. 30 minutes after meals

Answer C is correct. This is because Nexium is a proton pump inhibitor that should be taken before meals. Answers A, B, and D are incorrect administration times for proton pump inhibitors like Nexium.

88. The doctor has ordered ranitidine (Zantac) for a client with erosive gastritis. The nurse should give the medication:

a. 30 minutes before meals

b. With each meal

c. In a single dose at bedtime

d. 60 minutes after meals

Answer B is correct. This is because Zantac (rantidine) is a histamine blocker that should be taken with meals for optimal effect. Note however that Tagamet (cimetidine) is a histamine blocker that can be given in one dose at bedtime. Answers A and D are incorrect as neither of these drugs should be given before or after meals.

89. A client with gallstones and obstructive jaundice is experiencing severe itching. The doctor has ordered cholestyramine (Questran) and the client requested

information as to how this medication works. Which of the following statement is the best response a nurse can give?

a. "It binds with bile acids and is excreted in bowel movements with stool"

b. "It blocks histamine, thereby reducing the allergic response"

c. "It decreases the amount of bile in the gallbladder"

d. "It inhibits the enzyme responsible for bile excretion"

Answer A is correct. Questran works by binding the bile acid in the GI tract and eliminating it. This reduces the itching sensation associated with jaundice. Answers B, C, and D are incorrect as they are not answers as to how the medication works to decrease itching.

90. The nurse is looking after a client who abuses narcotics. The client is exhibiting a respiratory rate of 10 and dilated pupils. Which medication should the nurse expect to administer?

a. Chlordiazepoxide (Librium)

b. Haloperidol (Haldol)

c. Meperidine (Demerol)

d. Naloxone (Narcan)

Answer D is correct. The nurse should expect to administer Narcan. This is because the client is exhibiting signs of respiratory depression from the use of narcotics and therefore requires an antagonist to reverse the effects. Answer A and B are incorrect as these are antianxiety and antipsychotic medications, not narcotic-reversal drugs. Answer C is incorrect because Demerol is a narcotic that would only increase the adverse effects that the client is experiencing.

91. The client with urinary tract infection is placed on Furadantin. He may also receive ascorbic acid. The rationale to use this additional medication is to:

a. Promote tissue repair
b. Fortify mucosal repair
c. Alkalinize the urine
d. Acidify the urine

Answer D is correct. The antimicrobial activity of Furadantin is more effective in an acid urine. Because of this, ascorbic acid or vitamin C is used to acidify the urine. Answers A, B, and C are incorrect.

92. The nurse is about to instruct client about phenytoin sodium (Dilantin). Which information would be most important to teach the client as to why the drug should not be stopped abruptly?

a. A hypoglycemic reaction can develop

b. Heart block can develop

c. Status epilepticus can develop

d. The client can develop a physical dependence over time

Answer C is correct. A sudden discontinuation of seizure medication can cause status epilepticus to occur. This disorder is life threatening and it is therefore crucial that the client is informed about this. Answers A, B, and D are incorrect because these are not correct statements about the medication.

93. The physician orders dopamine for a client with left ventricular failure and a high pulmonary capillary wedge pressure (PCWP) to improve ventricular function. The nurse knows that the medication is having its intended effect when:

a. Blood pressure decreases

b. Blood pressure rises

c. Cardiac index falls

d. PCWP rises

Answer B is correct. The dopamine is having a desired effect when blood pressure rises. This is because it will cause vasoconstriction peripherally, but increase renal perfusion and the blood pressure will rise. Answer A is incorrect as it is the opposite of B. Answer C is also incorrect because the cardiac index will rise. Answer D is likewise incorrect because the PCWP should decrease.

94. The physician has prescribed a Becloforte (beclomethasone) inhaler two puffs twice a day for a client with asthma. The nurse should instruct the client to report:

a. A sore throat

b. Changes in mood

c. Difficulty in sleeping

d. Increased weight

Answer A is correct. This is because clients on steroid medications, including beclomethasone, can develop adverse side effects such as oral infections with candida albicans. Both a sore throat and white patches on the oral mucosa are symptoms of candida albicans and must therefore be reported immediately. Answers B, C, and D are incorrect because increased weight, difficulty sleeping, and changes in mood are all expected side effects of the medication.

95. The nurse visits a home client with hypertension who has been maintained on a daily dose of methyldopa (Aldomet). The client informs the nurse that they have been experiencing symptoms of lethargy and drowsiness. The appropriate nursing intervention would be to:

a. Ask the physician to order a different antihypertensive
b. Explain to the client that these are expected side effects
c. Report the negative side effects to the physician to have the dose reduced
d. Suggest that the client take the medication at bedtime and to reevaluate next time

Answer D is correct. These side effects may be present with this drug but can be alleviated if the drug is taken in the evening. Taking one dose in the evening can often minimize the sedation. The nurse should nevertheless report the side effects to the physician and follow up with the client. Answers A, B, and C are incorrect.

96. The mother of a client contacts the clinic informing that nurse that her daughter cannot swallow the capsule because it is too large. The nurse finds that the medication is a capsule marked *SR*. The nurse should instruct the mother to:

a. Call the pharmacist and request an alternative preparation of the medication
b. Crush the medication and administer it with 8 oz. of liquid
c. Open the capsule and mix the medication with ice cream
d. Stop the medication and inform the physician at the follow-up visit

Answer A is correct. *SR* stands for sustained release and these medications cannot be altered. The mother should therefore be instructed to request an alternative preparation of the medication from the pharmacist. Answers B and C are incorrect because crushing or opening the capsule is not allowed. Answer D is also incorrect as it is not necessary to notify the doctor immediately.

97. The client with rheumatoid arthritis has been placed on aspirin gr. xx TID and prednisone 10 mg BID for 2 years. The most important assessment the nurse should make is whether the client has experienced:

a. Blurred vision
b. A decreased sense of appetite
c. Headaches
d. Tarry stools

Answer D is correct. This is because aspirin impedes clotting by blocking prosta-glandin synthesis. This can lead to bleeding. A common side effect of the medication Prednisone is gastric irritation, which can likewise lead to bleeding. Tarry stools indicate bleeding in the upper GI system which should be immediately reported. Answers A, B, and D are incorrect. Although these should also be noted and reported, they are not the most important assessment for the nurse to make and are therefore incorrect.

98. A client scheduled for disc surgery informs the nurse that she frequently uses the herbal supplement kava-kava (piper methysticum). The nurse should immediately report this to the doctor because kava-kava:

a. Depresses the immune system, so infection is more of a problem

b. Eliminates the need for antimicrobial therapy following surgery

c. Increases the effects of anesthesia and post-operative analgesia

d. Increases urinary output, so a urinary catheter will be needed post-operatively

Answer C is correct. The herbal kava-kava can increase the effects of anesthesia and post-operative analgesia. Answers A, B, and D are incorrect because they are not related to the use of kava-kava.

99. The physician has ordered several medications including Beta Blocker Atenolol for a client with Congestive Heart Failure. The client requested information as to how this medication works. Which of the following statement is the best response a nurse can give?

a. "It causes vasodilation of coronary vessels"

b. "It increases the heart rate and forces contraction"

c. "It decreases the heart rate and forces contraction"

d. "It reduces myocardial oxygen demands"

Answer C is correct. Beta blockers decrease the heart rate and force contraction, thereby reducing vasoconstriction by antagonizing Beta receptors in the myocardium and vasculature. Answers A and D are incorrect as they refer to the action of nitrates and Calcium Channel Blockers such as Diltiazem. Answer B is also incorrect because it is the opposite of Answer C and therefore untrue.

100. A client with a detached retina has just been admitted and surgery has been scheduled. The nurse knows that the pre-op ophthalmic medication most likely to be ordered for the client will be:

a. Atropine sulfate

b. Carbamylcholine

c. Pilocarpine

d. Timolol maleate

Answer A is correct. This is because the medications used pre-op to widely dilate the pupil are Mydriatic drugs. Both Atropine sulfate and Epinephrine HCI are commonly used. Answer B and C are incorrect because these are miotics used for certain types of lens implants and glaucoma. Answer D is also incorrect because Timolol maleate is a beta blocker used for glaucoma.

101. A client is about to be discharged with an order for bishydroxycoumarin (Dicumarol). Which instructions should be included in the teaching plan?

a. The client should shave with an electric razor

b. The client should take the medication prior to eating

c. It is for the physician to teach the client about the medication

d. If the client misses a doe, he should take a double dose next time

Answer A is correct. The medication Dicumarol is an anticoagulant drug and because of this, one of the dangers is bleeding. Using a safety razor can lead to bleeding through cuts and the client should therefore use an electric razor. Answer B is incorrect because although the drug should be taken at the same time every day, there is no relation to meals. Answer C is incorrect and Answer D is also incorrect because, due to the danger of bleeding, missed doses should not be made up.

Cardiovascular System

Section 1: Introduction to the Cardiovascular System

The cardiovascular system is made up of the heart and blood vessels - it has the crucial responsibility of transporting oxygen and nutrients to the body's organ systems. It is therefore vitally important to spend enough time reviewing the diseases that can affect the cardiovascular system, along with how they are treated in your preparation for the NCLEX. On top of this, it is also essential to practice applying your knowledge with multiple practice questions. This concise preparation guide will cover the key points that you will need to know to be successful in the cardiovascular portion of your NCLEX test.

The guide begins with an outline of the topics and key facts on respiratory disorders that you need to remember for the exam. The list of subtopics can be seen on the contents page. In *Section 7* of this guide you can apply and test your knowledge with over 100 topic-specific practice questions. All answers to the questions are given, along with detailed rationales to further your knowledge and understanding of the topic.

Remember that ambition is the first step to success. The second step is action – hard work and determination. Purchasing this guide is an indication of your ambition, now it's time to get to work!

Best wishes,

Eva Regan

Section 2: Hypertension and Coronary Artery Disease

Hypertension

Key Points
- Blood pressure is the force of blood applied on the vessel walls.
- *Systolic pressure*: this is the pressure that occurs during the heart's contraction phase. The top number on a blood pressure reading monitors it.
- Diastolic pressure: this is the pressure that occurs during the heart's relaxation phase. The lower number on a blood pressure reading monitors it.
- Blood pressure higher than 140/90 indicates hypertension. For hypertension to be diagnosed, this pressure reading must be obtained on two different occasions.
- A reading higher than 130/85 is diagnosed as hypertension for clients with diabetes.
- Hypertension can be **primary/essential** – this develops with no apparent cause.
- Hypertension can be **secondary** – this develops due to another condition or illness. Examples of secondary causes: peripheral vascular disease, diabetes, renal disease, preeclampsia, and adrenal tumors.
- Malignant hypertension: can result in cerebral vascular accident or a myocardial infarction due to a greatly increased blood pressure.
- A number of medications can cause hypertension, such as non-steroidal anti-

inflammatory drugs (NSAID's), amphetamines, cocaine, bronchodilators.

Possible Signs and Symptoms
- Blurred vision
- Headache
- Dyspnea
- Signs of uremia if renal function is impaired.

A blood pressure larger than 200 mm Hg (systolic) and 150 mm Hg (diastolic) poses a threat to life.

Diagnosis

- The blood pressure cuff size affects the accuracy of the pressure reading. The cuff bladder size should be able to entirely circle the client's arm or thigh.
    - A cuff too small = falsely high pressure reading.
    - A cuff too large = falsely low pressure reading.
- Diagnosis includes a thorough analysis of the client's illness and stressor history, along with the medications that they have previously taken. Any underlying illness should be checked for via lab studies. For example, if serum corticoids and 17-ketosteroids are detected in urine, this is an indication of cushing's disease.
- Radiography study: used to confirm the presence of renal disease.
- X-Ray and CT scans: used to detect tumors.

- Electrocardiogram (ECG): used to monitor the involvement of the cardiovascular system.

Treatment/Management
- Reduction of stress
- Smoking cessation
- Exercise
- Low sodium diet. Low in fat and cholesterol
- Homocysteine levels can be reduced by folic acid.
- For client's those with a risk of coronary disease: Monounsaturated and polyunsaturated fats are recommended.

Medication
- If cholesterol is not lowered, medications can be prescribed, such as:
- Advicor (lovastation plus niacin)
- Caduet (amilodipine besylate plus atorvastatin calcium)
- Simvastatin (Zocor)
- Diuretics can be used for those who still have uncontrolled hypertension following a change diet and exercise. These lower lower blood pressure through diuresis
- Examples of non-potassium-sparing diuretics are hydrochlorothiazide (HCTZ) and Furosemide (Lasix). When taking these medications, the client should be assessed for hypokalemia signs.
- Potassium sparing diuretics decrease sodium ions.
- Antihypertensive medications can also be used to lower blood pressure. These block beta receptors. Examples: coreg (carvidilol) and

inderal (propanolol). The client should monitor their pulse rate due to the possibility of congestive heart failure and bradycardia.
- Calcium channel blockers (e.g. verapamil hydrochloride) can lower blood pressure by lowering calcium ions.
- Other drugs that can be used: Angiotensin Converting (e.g. Captopril (Procardia), enalpril (Vasotec)) and Angiotensin receptor blockers (e.g. Candesartan (Altacand), Iasartan (Cozaar)).

- Drugs can be used singularly or in combination with one another.

Coronary Artery Disease (CAD)

Key Points
- Ischemia occurs due to the narrowing of the coronary arteries that is usually caused by atherosclerosis.

ATHEROSCHLEROSIS & ARTERIOSCLEROSIS

- **Athero**sclerosis is a form of **arterio**sclerosis. It involves both cholesterol and triglyceride deposits and results in the narrowing of the blood vessels due to the overgrowth of smooth muscle cells – causing a reduction in blood flow to the heart, along with other organs.
- Arteriosclerosis involves the widening and hardening of the arterial walls.

Symptoms

- Decreased circulation (extremities).
- Irregular claudication
- Skin color changes
- Dizziness
- Headaches
- Loss of memory

Risk factors include: Obesity, smoking, diabetes, age.

Treatment

- Controlling the client's weight with a low fat and cholesterol diet
- Cessation of smoking
- Reduction of stress

Section 3: Cardiac Conduction System - Heart Block, ECG, Cardiac Dysrhythmias, & Angina Pectoris

The conduction system of the heart is made up of the sinoatrial (SA) node. This is situated at the junction of the superior vena cava and right atrium. This is the heart's main pacer that initiates contractions of the heart.

Situated near the interventricular septum is the atrioventricular (AV) node transmits impulse to his bundle.

Below is a representation of the heart's conduction system.

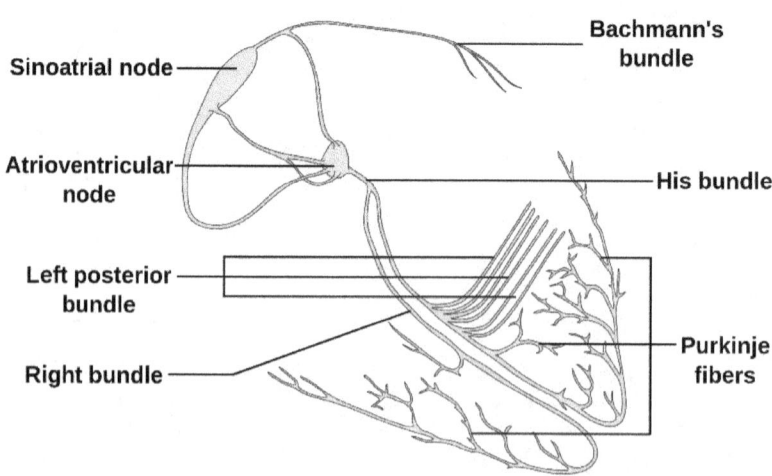

Heart Block

Key Points

- Caused due to structural changes in the cardiac conduction system, such as: coronary artery disease, infections of the heart, and tumors.
- **First degree AV block:** Transmissions of impulses from the SA node is slowed down. Heart beats consistently but the interval of the P-R is slowed down. Clients generally show no symptoms and all impulses ultimately reach the ventricles.
- **Second degree heart block:** Only some impulses reach the ventricles.
- **Third degree (complete) heart block:** No sinus impulses reach the ventricles. In this case, the SA and AV nodes beat individually. This can cause hypotension, seizures, and cardiac arrest.
- A heart block is detected using an electrocardiogram.

Toxicity to Medications

- Toxicity to medications can be linked with heart block. Examples of such medications are betablockers and calcium channel blockers.
- Clients that take betablockers should check their pulse rate and have their digitalis levels checked regularly.
- Digoxin (Digitalis) therapeutic levels: 0.9–1.2 ng/mL
- The client is determined toxic if Digoxin (Digitalis) is above 2.0 ng/mL.
- Symptoms of toxicity are often nausea and vomiting.
- The treatment for digitalis toxicity involves checking potassium levels, giving potassium orally or IV.

Medications (e.g. Isuprel or atropine) will often be given to increase the client's heart rate.

Conduction System Malfunction

- The malfunction of he conduction system is what generally leads to heart block.
- A pacing mechanism is usually implanted to assist with conduction.
- A demand pacemaker: A pacer that creates and impulse if the client's heart rate drops below a predetermined beats per minute.
- A set pacemaker: A pacer that entirely overrides the conduction system of the heart and generates a set impulse rate.
- Pacemakers are often used in combination with an internal defibrillation device.

Cardiac Monitoring with ECG

- The hearts electrical currents can be traced via ECG.
- Electrodes are placed on the client's chest, and they are connected via leads to an electrocardiograph machine.
- The leads consist of both positive and negative electrodes and common ECG machines are made up of 12 leads. 6 leads placed on the horizontal axis of the chest wall. The other leads are placed on limbs.
- The client should remain in a stationary position.
- The modified chest lead (MCL) system is generally used for continuous ECG readings, which includes three leads.

Reading an Electroriogram

- The P wave: atrial depolarization
- PR interval: The time it takes for the atria to depolarize and for the impulse to travel along the conduction system, reaching the Purkinje fibers.
- QRS complex: Measured from the beginning of the Q or R wave, to the end of the S wave. This gauges the contraction phase of the heart.
- T wave: repolarization of the heart

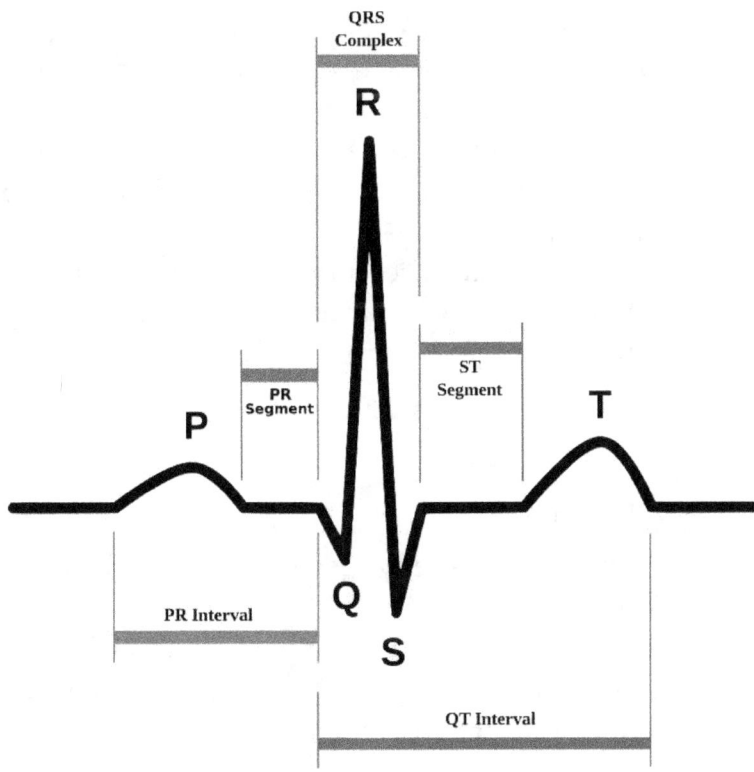

Measuring the heart rate: The heart rate is measured by monitoring and counting the number of PP/RR intervals on a 6 second ECG strip. The cardiac cycles and QRS complexes are counted and then multiplied by 10. This provides an accurate heart rate reading.

Normal rhythm: SA node, 60-100 regular beats per minute, consistent P wave, followed by a QRS complex.

Cardiac Dysrhythmias

Key Points

- The regular pacing capability of the heart is lost.
- Cardiac Dysrhythmias are classified by where they originate from.
- Can be either fatal or pose no danger.
- Tachydysrhythmias: heart rate greater than 100 beats per minute.
- Bradydysrhythmias: heart rate lower than 60 beats per minute. The client may experience dizziness and fainting.

Ventricular Tachycardia

- Rapid rhythm loss of a P wave.
- The heart rate is usually greater than 140-180 beats per minute.
- Lethal arrhythmia results in ventricular fibrillation.
- It is often linked with heart failure, hypotension, and hypomagnesium.

- **Treatment:** Oxygen and medication (e.g. Amiodarone (Cordarone), procainamide (Pronestyl)) that slows rate.

Ventricular Fibrilation

- The mechanism that is generally linked with cardiac arrest.
- Lack of pumping action in the heart.
- Blood is not sent to the brain and organs.
- If the condition is not corrected, asytole will be seen on the ECG.
- The client will start to lose consciousness and lose their pulse.
- Results in hypotension/lack of blood pressure.
  Treatment:

- Defibrillate the client, beginning with 200 Joules.
- Oxygen is provided, along with antidysrhythmic medications (e.g. epinephrine, amiodarone, procainamide).
- Cardiopulmonary resuscitation should be readied if cardiac arrest occurs.

Internal Pacemaker/Cardiac Defibrillator

- An internal pacemaker and cardioverter/defibrillator is a treatment of heart block, ventricular fibrillation, and dysrhythmias.
- These devices are attached with electric leads to the client's myocardium.
- The device delivers a shock to the heart to correct patterns when the client experiences ventricular tachycardia or fibrillation.

- The client with a internal pacemaker or defibrillator should be instructed to do the following:
- Avoid the elevation of the arms above head height for two weeks.
- Wear identification indicating the implantation of a pacemaker.
- Take their pulse.
- Refrain from applying pressure to the pacemaker.
- Refrain from near contact with electrical devices, especially microwaves.
- Move away from electromagnetic sources and people if beeping is heard coming from the internal defibrillator.
- Report any fainting, dizziness, rapid pulse rate changes etc.

Angina Pectoris

Key Points

- A disturbance the heart's balance and demand for oxygen.
- Causes a shortage of oxygen to the myocardium.
- Risk factors include: Hyperlipidemia, hypertension, smoking, obesity, diabetes, stress, and anemia.
- It is usually stimulated by a exertion, stress, anxiety, drugs, or alcohol.

Symptoms

- Pain is generally in the substernal to retrosternal area. The pain moves down through the left arm and is felt in the shoulder or jaw.
- Possible vomiting and nausea.

- Possible chest pain.
- Shortness and fatigue usually seen in older clients.

- An ECG generally shows depressions of the ST segment, along with inversions of the T wave.

Treatment

- Oxygen
- Nitroglycerine (sublingually, intravenously, or topically)
- Every five minutes, the client should take a nitroglycerine tablet sublingually, no more than three tablets. If the pain persists after three tablets, the client should go straight to a hospital.
- The client should replenish supplies of nitroglycerine regularly every 6 months.

Section 4: Myocardial Infarction, Congestive Heart Failure, Cardiogenic Shock

Myocardial Infarction

Key Points

- Disturbance of blood supply to the myocardium.
- Contributing factors include: arteriosclerosis, thrombus, emboli, hemorrhage.
- The heart becomes necrotic if blood circulation is not rapidly restored.
- Vasodilation can occur due to hypoxia from ischemia.
- The client can fall into cardiogenic shock due to acidosis which is linked with electrolyte imbalances.
- The left ventricle is the most frequent site for a myocardial infarction.

Signs and Symptoms

- Substernal pain/precordium pain for longer than fifteen minutes.
- Heavy pain down the left arm.
- Heavy pain in the neck and jaw.
- Shortness of breath
- Dizziness
- Nausea
- Vomiting
- Fall in blood pressure
- Rise in heart rate
- Rise in respiratory rate

Diagnosis

- Monitoring of the ECG and cardiac profile consisting of cardiac enzymes.
- Monitoring of white blood cell count, blood urea nitrogen, and sedimentations rate are other useful tests that can offer a better analysis of the condition that the client is in.
- Serum enzymes used to make a diagnosis: creatine kinase (CKMB), CRP, and LDH, troponin T and 1.
- CKMB increases quickly when there is a disturbance with the myocardium.
- Troponin T and 1 are utilized to measure the magnitude of the attack. They can be elevated for up to 2 weeks after a myocardium attack.

Management and Treatment

- Monitoring blood pressure.
- Monitoring oxygen levels.
- Monitoring pulmonary artery wedge pressures.
- Dopamine for rapid fall in blood pressure.
- Pain relief medications such as morphine sulfate IV.
- Medications to vasodilate the coronary vessels.
- Thrombolytics (e.g. streptokinase).
- Small and regular meals – low in fat, sodium, and cholesterol.
- Fluid and fiber to avoid constipation.
  Post Myocardial Infarction:

- Regular exercise
- Cessation of smoking
- Limited caffeine intake
- Sexual activity can be resumed in 6 weeks
- Medications clients will generally be discharged on: aspirin, enoxaparin (Lovenox), clopidogrel (Plavix).

Exercise Electrocardiography

- Assists in determining the heart's functioning during exercise.
- Prior to the test, the client must only eat a light meal and not smoke or consume caffeine.
1. The client is firstly given an ECG assessment.
2. The client engages in light exercise, such as walking on a treadmill.
3. The client is asked to inform the cardiologist of any chest pain or breath shortness.
4. The client continues until the either the maintenance of a rapid heart rate is reached, any signs of abnormalities are seen on the ECG, or ST depressions are noted on the ECG.
- The client stays in the unit for up to 2 hours following the test to make sure there are no indications of hypotension or cardiac dysrhythmias.

Echocardiography

- A non-invasive test used to determine the ventricle size, valve functionality, and heart size.
- The test generally takes 30 to 60 minutes.
- A more invasive method is a transesophageal echocardiography which assesses the structures of the heart.

Cardiac Catheterization

- Used to discover blockages that are linked with myocardial infarction.
- Requires signed consent.
- The nurse should: assess client's allergies to iodine/shellfish, assess renal function, ensure the

client is on a bed rest for up to 8 hours after the procedure, ensure pressure is kept on the access site for five minutes following the procedure, check distal pulses after procedure.

Percutaneous Transluminal Coronary Angioplasty and Stent Placement

- Relieves chest pain in many clients, especially those with non-calcified lesions.
- A catheter is inserted whilst the physician visualizes he coronary vessels. Plaque is pushed into the vessels using a balloon.
- A stent (stainless steel mesh tube) may be placed following the balloon.
- To prevent restenosis, the tube is inserted after angioplasty.
- The procedure is complete when 50 percent or more of the vessel is indicated to be open via angiography.
- IV of heparin is given, and sometimes Nitroglycerin or sublingual nifedipine to prevent myocardium spasms.

Coronary Artery Bypass Grafting (CABG)

- The physician may perform CABG surgery when the client fails to respond to coronary artery occlusion. This decision is made of result of the cardiac catheterization.

The signs that indicate when a CABG is necessary:

- Angina with larger than 50 percent left anterior descending artery blockage.

- Two vessels rigorously blocked, or three vessels that are somewhat blocked.
- Myocardium ischemia.
- Acute myocardium infarction.
- The clients requires intensive care following the procedure.
- Clients may experience nightmares and depressions following the surgery.
- Cardiac rehabilitation is generally needed following the procedure.

Congestive Heart Failure

Key Points

- The heart is unable to meet the body's oxygen requirements.
- **Cardiac output:** the volume of blood that is pumped within one minute. (stroke volume multiplied by heart rate).
- **Ejection fraction:** Stroke volume divided by end diastolic blood volume. A heart that is healthy has an ejection fraction of 50% to 70%.
- **Preload:** The stretch amount needed for blood to be forced out of the ventricle from the end of the diastole.
- **Afterload:** The force needed for blood volume ejection.
- If overstretching of the heart occurs, its ability to recoil is lost and the heart will eventually fail. This is when congestive heart failure occurs.

Signs

- Signs of fluid retention should be monitored by the nurse. Left sided congestive heart failure happens when fluid backs into the lugs. It is indicated by blood tinged sputum and rales.
- Right sided failure happens when there is peripheral edma, fatigue, and asites as a result of blood backing into the periphery.

Diagnosis

- Assessing symptoms and signs
- Assessing cardiac function
- ECG, blood pressure etc. can be used to evaluate the client's cardiac function.

Treatment

- Diuretics
- Inotropes
- Low sodium diet
- Medications to improve cardiac contractility:
- IV nitroprusside
- Milrinone (Primacor)
- Nitroglycerine nesiritide (natrecor)
- Medications to support cardiac function:
- Angiotensin receptor blockers (ARBs)
- Angiotensin-converting enzyme (ACE) inhibitors
- Beta blockers

Cardiogenic Shock

- **Types of shock:** Cardiogenic shock, vasogenic/neurogenic shock, and hypovolemic shock.
- Cardiogenic shock happens as a result of the heart failing to pump enough to perfuse the tissues sufficiently. The cause of this shock could be due to myocardial infarction, pericarditis, congestive heart failure, and cardiac tamponade, along with other cardiac complications.
- Hypovolemic shock happens as result of a lack of blood flow which is unable to maintain blood pressure. The result of this is a decrease in oxygen received by the major organs.
- Vasogenic/neurogenic shock occurs due to brain or spinal cord trauma.

Symptoms

- Tachycardia
- Tachypnea
- Hypotension
- Frothy, pink-tinged sputum
- Restlessness
- Orthopnea
- Oliguria

If cardiogenic shock is not identified early, there is a high rate of mortality.

Treatment:

- Oxygen therapy
- Morphine sulfate for pain relief

To reduce the preload:

- Diuretics
- Nitroglycerin

Section 5: Aneurysms, Inflammatory Heart Diseases

<u>Aneurysms</u>

Key Points

- The ballooning of an artery is known as an aneurysm.
- Poses a high risk of rupture and hemorrhage.
- Can be a result of arteriosclerosis, or secondary to hypertension
  There are a number of types of aneurysms:

- **Fusiform** that impacts the artery's entire circumference.
- **Saccular** that affects just one portion of the artery.
- **Dissecting** which is bleeding into the vessel's wall.

Signs and Symptoms

- Pain in the lower back
- Client feels as if their heart were beating in their abdomen

Diagnosis

- Ultrasound
- Arteriogram
- Abdominal x-rays
- A aneurysm of 5 centimeters or larger may be scheduled for surgery

Inflammatory Heart Diseases

Infective Endocarditis

- Generally due to bacterial infections or collagen diseases.
- Possibly related to cancer metastasis
- Results in damage of the heart (cardiac decompensation)

Signs and Symptoms

- Shortness of breath
- Chest pain
- Fatigue
- Distended neck veins
- Cardiac Murmur

Treatment

- Antibiotics to treat underlying cause
- Oxygen therapy
- Anti-inflammatory drugs
- Possibly valve replacement if valve is rigorously damaged

Pericarditis

Key Points

- A pericardium inflammation condition.
- The pericardium is the heart's membrane sac.

Signs and Symptoms

- Breathing difficulty
- Chest pain
- Fever
- Right sided congestive heart failure
- Pericardial friction rub is generally seen
- An elevated white blood cell count might be seen
- A likely ECG is an ST segment and T wave increase
- Pericardial effusion is frequently seen in the echocardiogram

Treatment

- Nonsteroidal anti-inflammatory medication for pain relief.
- Possible pericardiocentesis.
- Pericardium might be removed in severe cases.

Peripheral Vascular Disease

Key Points

- A number of diseases that affect the arteries and veins.
- Peripheral arterial disease is the most common.
- Frequently results in disease of the kidney, amputations, and extremity ulcers.

Signs and Symptoms

- Fall in pulse
- Decrease in strength

- Leg cramps
- Coldness and swelling of the extremity

Treatment

- Blood flow restoration to the extremity.
- As a final resort, sever the sympathetic ganglia via sympathectomy.
- Vasodilating drugs.
- Femoropopliteal bypass graft may be made.
- Possible amputation is circulation is not restored.

Varicose Veins & Thrombophlebitis

- **Varicose veins** are present when there is a collapse of the valves that push blood back to the heart.
- Blood pools in the veil that can cause blood clots and eventually result in a pulmonary emboli.
- **Thrombophlebitis** occurs as a results of an inflamed vein – this causes a clot. The saphenous vein is the most frequently affected vein.
- To assess deep vein thrombi, Homan's sign is used. **Treatment:**

- Leg compression, anticoagulants (heparin, enoxaparin, or sodium warfarin).
- Antibiotics if cellulitis is present.
- Antithrombolitic stockings

Raynaud's Phenomenon

Key Points

- Exposure to cold causes vascular vasospasms.

- Women more commonly affected.
- **Management:** Preventing cold exposure, cessation of smoking, and vasodilators.

Buerger's Disease

Key Points

- Artery and vein spasms in the lower extremities.
- Results in the formation of blood clots and the vessel destruction.
- **Symptoms:** Extremity pallor, cyanosis, parethesia.
- **Management:** Buerger-Allen exercises, oxygenation, vasodilators, cessation of smoking.

Section 6: Key Terms & Diagnostic Exams

Below you will find a summary of the key terms that you will need to be knowledgeable of, along with the main diagnostic exams that are used to detect cardiovascular problems.

Key Terms

- Aneurysms
- Angina pectoris
- Angioplasty
- Atherosclerosis
- Buerger's disease
- Cardiac catheterization
- Cardiac tamponade
- Cardiopulmonary resuscitation
- Cholesterol
- Conduction system of the heart
- Congestive heart failure
- Coronary artery bypass graft
- Defibrillation
- Diastole
- Electrocardiogram
- Heart block
- Hypertension
- Implantable cardioverter
- Myocardial infarction
- Pacemaker
- Raynaud's phenomenon
- Systole
- Thrombophlebitis

- Varicose veins
- Ventricular fibrillation
- Ventricular tachycardia

Key Diagnostic Exams

- Cardiac catheterization
- Cardiac CTA
- Cardiac profile
- Central venous pressure monitoring
- Chest x-ray
- Clotting studies
- Complete blood count
- Doppler studies
- Dye studies for cardiac functions
- Echocardiogram
- Electrophysiologic studies
- Exercise Tolerance Test
- Fluoroscopy
- MRI
- Oxygen saturation levels
- Serum cholesterol and triglycerides
- Serum electrolytes
- Thallium scans
- Ultrasonography
- Vital signs

Section 7: Cardiovascular System Questions and Rationales

1. An order for furosemide is made for a client with hypertension. Which of the following lab findings should be reported to the physician?

a. Phosphorus 2.5 mEq/L

b. Calcium 9.4 mg/dl

c. Magnesium 2.4 mEq/L

d. Potassium 1.8 mEq/L

Answer D is correct. The furosemide poses a risk for the development of hypokalemia for the client. This is because this drug is a non-pottasium-sparing diuretic. Cardiac dysrhythmias may be cause by a low potassium level. Answers A, B, and C are incorrect – these are normal levels.

2. A diagnosis of heart block has been made for a client who has been admitted. Which of the following is the pacemaker of the heart?

a. SA node

b. AV node

c. Purkinje fibers

d. Bundle of His

Answer A is correct. The SA node is the pacemaker of the heart. The impulse travels from the SA node to the AV node on to the right and left bundle branches and ultimately to the Purkinje fibers. Answers B, C, and D incorrect.

3. **Nitroprusside (Nitropress) is being treated in a client. What should the nurse be aware of about this medication?**

a. It is a non–potassium-sparing diuretic

b. It should be protected from light

c. It decreases circulation to the extremities

d. It causes vasoconstriction

Answer B is correct. Light decreases the effectiveness of nitroglycerine preparations, therefore it should be shielded from light. Nitroprusside is not a diuretic, therefore answer A is incorrect. Answer C is incorrect because it does not reduce circulation to the extremities. Answer D is incorrect because nitroprusside is a not a vasoconstrictor, but a vasodilator.

4. **A hacking cough is developed by a client that is being**

treated with lisinopril (Zestril). What should the nurse tell the client to do?

a. Report the problem to the doctor

b. Take half the dose to control the problem

c. Take cough medication to control the problem

d. Stop the medication

Answer A is correct. A hacking cough is a frequent side effect that should be reported to the doctor. Answer B is incorrect because an elevated blood pressure can be caused by halving the dose. Answer C is incorrect because any allergic reactions will be masked by taking cough medications. Answer D is incorrect because the client should report to the doctor immediately.

5. Constipation is developed by an elderly client who is taking digitalis. Which of the following might result for a client experiencing constipation taking digitalis:

a. Result in a lowered digitalis level

b. Result in an elevated digitalis level

c. Result in alterations in the sodium level

d. Result in tachycardia

Answer B is correct because taking digitalis can result in a rise in digitalis level. Answers A, C, and D are incorrect.

6. A myocardial infarction is suspected in a client. Which of the following diagnostic findings is most substantial?

a. LDH

b. Creatinine

c. Troponin

d. AST

Answer C is correct. Troponin is the most effective confirmation tool used to confirm the client has developed myocardial infarction. CKMB is also a lab value linked with myocardial infarction. Answer A is incorrect because an elevation of LDH is not associated with myocardial infarction, but with muscle trauma. Answer B is incorrect because renal function is indicated by creatinine level. Answer D is incorrect because the elevation of the AST is not associated with myocardial infarction, but with gallbladder, muscle inflammation, and liver disease.

7. Which of the following should a client with an

internally implanted defibrillator should be instructed to do?

a. Avoid driving a car

b. Report swelling at the site

c. Avoid eating food cooked in a microwave

d. Refrain from using a cellular phone

Answer B is correct. Swelling at the site of the implant should be reported for the client with an implanted defibrillator. Answers A, C, and D are incorrect because all of these can be done by the client. The client will likely be instructed to refrain from driving for three months, to use a cell phone in the right hand, and not be close to a microwave whilst cooking.

8. Cardiac catheterization is scheduled for a client. Which of the following should the nurse do following the procedure?

a. Assess the urinary output

b. Assess for allergy to iodine

c. Check pulses proximal to the site

d. Check to ensure that the client has a consent form signed

Answer A is correct. A decrease in renal function can be caused by the dye that is used in the procedure. Assessments of the renal function should be made and changes should be reported immediately. Answer B is incorrect because allergies should not be checked after the procedure, but should be checked prior to the procedure. Answer C is incorrect because pulses should not be checked proximal to the site, but distal to the site. Answer D is incorrect because the consent should be signed before the procedure.

9. Pain in the lower extremities is reported by a client with Buerger's disease. Which of the following is another name for Buerger's disease?

a. Pheochromocytoma

b. Thromboangiitis obliterans

c. Intermittent claudication

d. Kawasaki disease

Answer B is correct. Thromboangiitis obliterans is another name for Buerger's disease. Answer A is incorrect because it is an adrenal tumor. Answer C is incorrect because intermittent claudication is an extremity pain while walking. Answer D is incorrect - Kawasaki disease is an acute vasculitis which can cause a thoracic area aneurysm.

10. Which of the following does a client with an abdominal aneurysm commonly report:

a. A headache

b. Shortness of breath only during sleep

c. Difficulty voiding

d. Lower back pain

Answer D is correct. Lower back pain, nausea, and feeling as if their heartbeat is in their abdomen is often experienced by those with abdominal aneurysms. Answer A is incorrect because headaches are generally associated with cerebral aneurysm. Answer B is incorrect because breath shortness is not specific to sleep in abdominal aneurysm. Answer C is incorrect because this is not linked with abdominal aneurysm.

11. Following a coronary artery bypass graft, the client is admitted to the intensive care area. The nurse that is caring for the client controls the fluid volume status by monitoring the central venous pressure and a reading of 2 mm Hg is shown. Which of the following actions should be taken by the nurse?

a. Continue their care with no further action

b. Decrease the IV fluid with the protocol provided

c. Increase the rate of IV fluid with the protocol provided

d. Give furosemide (Lasix) as ordered

Answer C is correct. 8–12 mm Hg is a normal central venous pressure reading. A reading of 2 mm Hg is an indication of possible bleeding and loss of fluid. IV fluid should be administered as ordered. Answers A, B, and D are improper actions.

12. Diuretics and beta-blockers for a client with hypertension. Which of the following should the client do when taking beta-blockers?

a. Check their pulse rate daily

b. Refrain from operating heavy equipment such as a bulldozer

c. Allow six weeks for the medication to reach its optimal level

d. Increase their intake of potassium-rich foods

Answer A is correct. The client should be instructed to check their pulse daily. Answer B is incorrect because the client is allowed to operate heavy equipment whilst taking betablockers. Answer C is incorrect because the optimal levels of beta blockers are reached within days of starting the medication. It is unnecessary to increase potassium intake via food for diuretics that are not potassium sparing.

13. An order for furosemide (Lasix) to be taken by a client every morning. Which of the following foods contains the highest level potassium?

a. One-half cup of mashed potatoes

b. One baked potato

c. One-fourth cup of sweet potatoes

d. One cup of french-fried potatoes

Answer B is correct. Large quantities of potassium are found in the skin of a baked potato. Answers A, C, and D are incorrect because they contain lower amounts of potassium.

14. An order is made to reduce the amount of cholesterol in the diet for a client with hypercholesterolemia. Which of the following cooking oils contains the most cholesterol?

a. Safflower

b. Sunflower

c. Canola

d. Palm

Answer D is correct. Palm oil is are very high in cholesterol, and such oils pose a risk factor to coronary artery disease. Safflower and sunflower are recommended for clients with coronary artery disease, therefore answers A and B are incorrect. Canola oil contains less cholesterol and fat than palm oil, therefore answer D is incorrect.

15. To control their hypercholesterolemia, the client has been prescribed simvastatin (Zocor). Which of the following should the client be taught to do when taking the medication?

a. Have his liver enzyme assessed every six months

b. Take the medication with grapefruit juice

c. Take the medication in the morning for the best absorption

d. Inform the physician of any weakness or drowsiness

Answer A is correct. Liver enzymes should be assessed every six months, this is because simvastatin (Zocor) can cause damage to the liver. Answer B is incorrect because is should not be ingested with grapefruit juice. Simvastatin should be taken at nighttime for best absorption, therefore answer C is incorrect. Answer D is incorrect because weakness is not associated with this medication.

16. The client with hypertension has an order for lisinopril plus hydrochlorothiazide (HTCZ) (Zestorectic). Prior to their initial dose, the client should be taught to:

a. Stay in bed for 3 to 4 hours after taking the first dose

b. Check his pulse rate every day

c. Expect a fall in his cholesterol level within six weeks

d. Increase their intake of folic-acid–rich food such (e.g. orange juice)

Answer A is correct. Postural hypotension can be caused by Lisinopril (Zestril). The client should be taught to remain stationary for 3 to 4 hours following the first dose. To determine the effects of the medication, the client's blood pressure should be measured regularly. Answer B is incorrect because lisinopril does not directly affect the pulse rate. Lisinorpril does not decrease cholesterol levels, therefore answer C is incorrect. It is unnecessary to increase folic acid along with lisinopril, therefore answer D is incorrect.

17. There are adverse effects of angiotensin-converting agents. Which of the following should be reported to the doctor?

a. Postural dizziness

b. Occasional nausea

c. Persistent hacking cough

d. Pedal edema

Answer C is correct. An adverse effect that is often linked with angiotensin-converting agents is a hacking cough. This cough could be an indication of an allergy to the medication. Answer A is incorrect because dizziness may be experienced upon arising. Occasional nausea is not an adverse effect linked with angiotensin-converting agents, therefore answer B is incorrect. Answer D is incorrect because pedal edema is not linked with angiotensin-converting agents, but with the retention of fluid and peripheral vascular disease.

18. Nitroglycerine should be taken sublingually by a client with angina at the beginning of the initial signs of chest pain. Which of the following instructions should be given to the client:

a. Keep the medication in the brown bottle to preserve the strength of the medication.

b. Take one tablet every 10 minutes until the pain subsides.

c. If a burning sensation of the tongue occurs, stop the medication immediately.

d. Refill the supply of nitroglycerine every three months.

Answer A is correct. The medication is deteriorated by light, therefore it should be kept in a brown bottle. The client can take a pill each 5 minutes (three doses), therefore Answer B is incorrect. They should go to the emergency department if the pain does not subside. Answer C is incorrect because a burning feeling is normal. The supply of nitroglycerine should be refilled every 6 months, therefore answer D is incorrect.

19. **A permanent pacemaker has been implanted in a client with heart block (fourth degree). What should the client with a pacemaker avoid?**

a. Using a cellular phone

b. Wearing a pager

c. Having a magnetic resonance imaging test

d. Traveling by airplane

Answer C is correct. Magnetic resonance imaging testing should not be given to those with a pacemaker or an internal defibrillator. Answers A and B are incorrect because such devices can be used by clients with a pacemaker, provided they are used on the opposite side of the pacemaker. The client is able to travel by airplane, therefore answer D is incorrect.

20. A client is taking digitalis (Lanoxin). Which of the following breakfast selections would be best for the client?

a. A bagel with jelly and a coffee

b. Bran muffin, orange juice, and coffee

c. Bacon and egg on toast and a coffee

d. Ham-and-cheese biscuit and a coffee

Answer B is correct. The client taking digitalis (Lanoxin) can avoid toxicity by increasing the amount of fiber in his diet. The bran muffin and orange juice offer the highest amounts of fiber. The orange juice provides potassium, but to avoid toxicity this should be consumed moderately. The other options are lower in fiber, therefore answers A, C, and D are incorrect.

21. Which of the following symptoms will be experienced if the client becomes toxic to their digitalis:

a. Tachycardia

b. Nausea and vomiting

c. Hypotension

d. Diarrhea

Answer B is correct. Nausea, vomiting, and brachycardia are signs of digitalis toxicity. Answer A is incorrect because they will not experience tachycardia, but will experience brachycardia. Answer C is incorrect because although hypotension can occur, it is not a sign of toxicity. A client with diarrhea is not likely to be toxic, therefore Answer D is incorrect.

22. A client with a history of cardiac disease is having an ECG tracing. Which of the following areas should the negative lead be placed?

a. The anterior right leg of the client

b. The left chest at the second intercostal space

c. The left chest at the apex of the heart

d. The right chest at the second intercostal space

Answer D is correct. The negative lead/white lead is positioned on the client's right side at the second intercostal space. The other areas are not where the negative lead is placed, therefore answers A, B, and D are incorrect.

23. A seven-week-old patient with aortic stenosis who has an

order for aortic stenosis is having their pulse checked. A pulse rate of 82 beats per minute is found for the client. Which action is most appropriate?

a. Administer the medication and recheck the pulse rate 30 minutes later

b. Administer the medication and document the pulse rate

c. Contact the physician prior to administering the medication

d. Withhold the medication and document the finding

Answer C is correct. A pulse rate of below than 100 beats per minute in the infant should be reported to the physician. The nurse should not give the medication if the pulse rate is below 100 beats per minute, therefore answers A and B are incorrect. The nurse should report this finding, therefore answer answer d is incorrect.

24. Following a car accident, the client is admitted to the emergency room. Frequent premature ventricular contractions are revealed by ECG. Which of the following medications is generally used to treat premature ventricular contractions?

a. Atropine sulfate (Atropine)

b. Epinephrine bitartrate (Epinephryl)

c. Enoxaparin (Lovenox)

d. Amiodarone (Cordarone)

Answer D is correct. Amiodarone (Cordarone) can be used as a treatment for premature ventricular contractions. This drug will work to slow down the heart rate. Lidocaine and magnesium sulfate will also have the same effect. Atropine sulfate (Atropine) and Epinephrine bitartrate (Epinephryl) speed up the heart rate, therefore answers A and B are incorrect. Enoxaparin (Lovenox) is a heparin derivative that is used as an anticoagulant, therefore answer C is incorrect.

25. A client with ventricular fibrillation is admitted. Defibrillation should be started by shocking at what level?

a. 200 Joules

b. 360 Joules

c. 400 Joules

d. 600 Joules

Answer A is correct. When defibrillation is performed, three rapid consecutive shocks are given with the third shock at 360 Joules. Answer B is incorrect because only the third shock should be 360 Joules. 400 and 600 Joules are too high, therefor answers C and D are incorrect.

26. A client admitted with severe chest pain is being cared for by the nurse. What should the nurse's next action be after assessing the vital signs?

a. Administer morphine

b. Get ready to administer oxygen by mask

c. Prepare the defibrillator

d. Take a complete history from the client

Answer B is correct. When providing care for the client with chest pain, the nurse should be prepared to apply oxygen. Oxygen can be given to elevate the myocardium oxygenation. Answer A is incorrect because morphine can be only be administered after obtaining an order. It is unnecessary to defibrillate the client, therefore answer C is incorrect. A history of the client should be taken when the client is in a stable position, therefore answer D is incorrect.

27 Cardiac catheterization is scheduled for a client with arteriosclerosis. Which is the nurse's main responsibility before the procedure?

a. Give an explanation of the procedure to the client

b. Take the client's vital signs

c. Check the laboratory results for a prothrombin time

d. Obtain a permit for the examination

Answer B is correct. The main duty of the nurse is to obtain the vital signs. Answers A, C, and D are incorrect because the it is the doctor who has primary responsibility for giving an explanation of the procedure, obtaining a permit, and examining the laboratory results for a prothrombin time.

28. What should the nurse do following a client's cardiac catheterization where the femoral artery is utilized as the access vessel?

a. Assess for allergies to iodine

b. Assess the pedal pulse in the operative leg

c. Tell the client to refrain from drinking liquids

d. Explain the need to flex and extend the leg

Answer B is correct. A clot might be present, therefore checking the pulse in the procedure extremity is crucial. A decreased pulse rate will be seen when a clot is present. Answers A and C are incorrect because assessing for allergies and withholding fluids should be done before the procedure. To increase the secretion of dye by the kidneys, the client should drink more after the procedure. The client should keep their leg straight, therefore answer D is incorrect.

29. A client is admitted two weeks following the start of chest pain. Which of the following laboratory tests is most indicative of myocardial infarction?

a. Troponin level

b. Creatine kinase (CK-MB)

c. Lactic acid dehydrogenase (LDH)

d. Blood urea nitrogen (BUN)

Answer A is correct. Levels of Troponin can remain increased for up to two weeks. Answer B is incorrect because if the client had a myocardial infarction two weeks ago, the creatine kinase (CK-MB) will have likely been restored to normal. Answers C and D are incorrect because although they can be increased with a myocardial infarction, they are not particular to this condition.

30. After a coronary artery bypass graft, a client returns to the intensive care unit. The client suddenly begins to experience shortness of breath with muffled heart sounds. The client's blood pressure is 90/40, and the pulse rate is 110 beats per minute. Which of the following is the most

appropriate initial action:

a. Recheck the vital signs

b. Administer pain medication

c. Check the mediastinal tube for drainage

d. Decrease the intravenous flow rate

Answer C is correct. Cardiac tamponade or fluid around the heart is indicated by muffled heart sounds and an absence of drainage from the mediastinal tube. The physician should be informed of this immediately. Answer A is incorrect because this wastes crucial time. Answer B is incorrect because there is nothing to indicate that pain medication is needed. This could also decrease the client's blood pressure. Decreasing the intravenous flow rate can cause additional shock, therefore answer D is incorrect.

31. A client is recovering from a myocardial infarction. Which breakfast cereal option is the best for recovery?

a. Instant-cooking cereals

b. Raisin Bran

c. Cocoa Puffs

d. Puffed rice

Answer D is correct. Puffed rice, puffed contains less sodium than the other choices, therefore answers A, B, and C are incorrect.

32. An order for milrinone (Primacor) is made for a client with congestive heart failure. What should the nurse do if the doctor decides to check the BNP?

a. Slow the rate of the Primacor infusion

b. Administer a diuretic prior to checking the BNP

c. Stop the Primacor for 2 hours prior to the test

d. Continue the Primacor as ordered

Answer C is correct. Primacor should be stopped 2 hours prior to the test, to ensure accurateness of the BNP laboratory test. Answers A, B, and D incorrect as they are not the correct actions to take.

33. A prescription for sodium warfarin (Coumadin) is provided to a client who has been discharged. What should the nurse teach the client to do?

a. Increase the amount of fiber in the diet to avoid constipation

b. Take the medication only with water

c. Consume green vegetables at least three times per week

d. Administer the medication in the abdomen with a tuberculin syringe

Answer A is correct. When taking sodium warfarin, constipation can lead to an elevated level. The absorption of this medication can be affected. Answer B is incorrect because the medication can be taken with a range of liquids. Answer C is incorrect because the client should not eat more than one serving of green/leafy vegetables each week. Answer D is incorrect because sodium is not administered by injection, but is taken orally.

34. A 50-year-old woman is admitted to the emergency room and reports indigestion and back and shoulder pain. She has taken a number of antacids for the previous two days without relief of the symptoms. Which of the following actions would be most appropriate:

a. Find out if the client if has a history of gastric ulcers

b. Obtain the client's vital signs and contact the physician

c. Let the client to rest undisturbed

d. Obtain a history to rule out a hiatal hernia

Answer B is correct. These symptoms culd indicate a myocardial infarction. Obtaining the vital signs and reporting to the physician will let the doctor make an order for laboratory tests and an ECG to rule out an myocardial infarction. Answers A, C, and D are incorrect because they waste valuable time.

35. A client is receiving Coumadin (warfarin sodium has a Protime level of 44 seconds). Which of the following should the nurse anticipate an order for:

a. Physostigmine

b. AquaMEPHYTON

c. Ropivacaine

d. Methimazole

Answer B is correct. AquaMEPHYTON is the alternative name for vitamin K. Physostigmine is Antilirium that is an anticholinesterase medication which is used to reverse the effects of diazepam (Valium), therefore answer A is incorrect. Answer C is incorrect because ropivacaine is Naropin, a medication that is used as a local anesthetic. Answer D is incorrect because methimazole is Tapazole, a medication that is used to treat hypothyroidism.

36. A diagnosis of congestive heart failure is made for a client that has been admitted. Which of the following findings indicates a diagnosis of left-sided congestive heart failure?

a. Pitting edema 3+

b. Tachycardia

c. Ascites

d. Fatigue

Answer B is correct. Tachycardia and coughing with pink-tinged sputum are symptoms of left-sided congestive heart failure. Answers A and C are incorrect because they are symptoms of right-sided congestive heart failure. Fatigue is not particular to the diagnosis of left-sided congestive failure, therefore answer D is incorrect.

37. Which of the following statements from a client would cause suspicion for sacular abdominal aortic aneurysm by the nurse?

a. "I sometimes have indigestion when lying down."

b. "I feel tired and shortness of breath with minimal

exertion."

c. "I frequently have pulsating sensations in my abdomen."

d. "I have severe pain radiating down my left arm."

Answer B is correct. The presence of pulsation in the abdomen is a frequent complaint in clients with an abdominal aortic aneurysm. Indigestion when lying down is an indication of gastroesophageal reflux disorder (GERD), therefore answer A is incorrect. Answer C is incorrect because symptoms of fatigue and shortness of breath with minimal exertion could be an indication of congestive heart failure. Answer D is incorrect because radiating left arm pain can be an indication of a myocardial infarction.

38. The client returns from surgery following a coronary artery bypass graft with a mitral valve replacement. Which medication will be ordered for the client who has a metal valve replacement?

a. Sodium warfarin (Coumadin)

b. Chlorothiazide (Diuril)

c. Clonidine HCl (Catapres)

d. Propranolol (Inderal)

Answer A is correct. Lifelong anticoagulant therapy with drugs such as sodium warfarin (Coumadin) are required for clients with a metallic valve replacement. Answer B is incorrect because chlorothiazide (Diuril) is a diuretic. Clonidine HCl (Catapres) is an antihypertensive, therefore answer C is incorrect. Answer D is incorrect because propranolol (Inderal) is a beta-blocker that is used for hypertension.

39. A diagnosis of intermittent claudication is made for a client with peripheral vascular disease. Which of the following actions by the nurse would assist the client to relieve symptoms of intermittent claudication?

a. Encourage the use of a heating pad to the effected leg

b. Use antithrombolytic stockings as ordered

c. Massage the effected extremity

d. Encourage the client to ambulate

Answer B is correct. Using antithrombolytic stockings will help with supporting muscles and blood vessels and reduces blood pooling. A heating pad can result in burning for the client with peripheral vascular disease, therefore answer A is incorrect. Massaging the extremity can result in pulmonary embolism, therefore answer C is incorrect. Ambulation elevates the pain of the client, therefore answer D is incorrect.

40. A client has a femoral popliteal bypass graft. Which of the following instructions should be given to the client before discharge:

a. Rest in high Fowler's position

b. Avoiding crossing the legs at the ankles

c. Check the radial pulse rate daily

d. Keep the procedural leg straight

Answer D is correct. A client with a femoral popliteal bypass graft should be instructed to keep the procedural leg as straight as they can. Bending or crossing the leg at the knee can hinder circulation and shut the grafted vessel. The client should rest in a semi-Fowler's position, therefore answer A is incorrect. Answer B is incorrect because the client can not cross the legs at the knee, but can cross their legs at the ankles. Answer C is incorrect because the radial pulse does not need to be checked daily. The pedal and posterior tibial pulses can show decreased blood flow.

41. Following a myocardial infarction, which of the following instructions should be given to the client when being discharged:

a. You should take nitroglycerine at the first signs of chest pain.

b. You can begin having intercourse when you can climb three flights of stairs without experiencing breathlessness.

c. You can take sildenafil (Viagra) for erectile dysfunction.

d. You should walk at least three miles every day to increase cardiac output.

Answer A is correct. Nitroglycerine should be taken at the first sign of chest pain for a client who has experienced a myocardial infarction. To treat angina pain, the client can take three sublingual tablets. The client should go to the hospital if the pain continues. The client can begin having intercourse when they can climb one flight of stairs breathlessly, therefore answer B is incorrect. Viagra should not be taken within 24 hours of taking a nitrite (e.g. nitroglycerine), therefore answer C is incorrect. Answer D is incorrect because the three miles per day is too excessive for the client, they should be involved in a 'step' program that progressively increases physical activity.

42. A client is admitted with potential thrombophlebitis. Which of the following actions should most important?

a. Assess using Homan's sign

b. Schedule a Doppler study for the client

c. Ask the client to stay in bed

d. Apply a moist heat pad to the extremity

Answer C is correct. The client should stay in bed to reduce the threat of a pulmonary embolus. Answer A is incorrect because Homan's sign is no longer used to gauge the client for the presence of thrombophlebitis because this assessment tool can result in the clot to dislodging and travelling to the lungs. Answer B is incorrect because the schedule for a Doppler study will be made by the doctor. Answer D is incorrect because applying a heat pad to the extremity will be ordered by the doctor once the client has been fully assessed.

43. What should the client with Raynaud's phenomena be taught to do?

a. Wear mittens when she is out in the cold

b. Keep the feet elevated while resting

c. Avoid caffeine intake

d. Drink warm liquids to loosen lung secretions

Answer A is correct. Raynaud's phenomena is a vascular spasm that happens due to exposure to cold. The hands are commonly affected, therefore wearing mittens will help with reducing the symptoms of Raynaud's phenomena. Answer B is incorrect because there is no association between keeping the feet elevated and the occurrence of Raynaud's phenomena. Caffeine intake is not linked with Raynaud's phenomena, therefore answer C is incorrect. Answer D is incorrect because Raynaud's phenomena is not a problem that is linked with lung disorders.

44. Buerger's disease is being treated in the client. What is an alternative name for Buerger's disease is:

a. Thrombophlebitis

b. Coronary thrombosis

c. Arteritis

d. Thromboangiitis obliterans

Answer D is correct. Buerger's disease occurs when spasms of the arteries and veins occur, mostly in the lower extremities. These spasms result in eventual destruction of the vessels due to the formation of blood clots. Thrombophlebitis is a blood clot that involves inflammation of the vein, therefore answer A is incorrect. Answer B is incorrect because coronary thrombosis is a coronary artery clot. Answer C is incorrect because arteritis is an inflammation of the arteries.

45. A client's central venous pressure is being monitored by the nurse. Which of the following positions would give

the most accurate measurement of the central venous pressure?

a. High Fowler's

b. Supine

c. Left Sims'

d. Prone

Answer B is correct. The nurse should put the client in a supine position to accurately assess the central venous pressure. The zero reference point on the manometer should be located at the fifth intercostal space, mid-axillary line/phlebostatic axis. Answers A, C, and D will not give a correct reading therefore they are incorrect.

46. Rosuvastatin (Crestor) is given to a client with a serum cholesterol of 275 mg/dl. Which of the following instructions should be given to the client?

a. Allow six months for the drug to take effect.

b. Report weakness of muscles to the physician.

c. Take the medication with fruit juice.

d. Ask the doctor to perform a complete blood count before starting the medication.

Answer B is correct. Muscle weakness is a sign of rhabdomyolysis, therefore the client taking antilipidemics should report weakness to the physician. Answer A is incorrect because the medication takes effect within one month of starting therapy. Answer C is incorrect because the medication should be taken with water. Answer D is incorrect because complete blood count should not be checked, but Liver function studies should be before beginning the medication.

47. A client with a hypertensive crisis has been admitted to the hospital. An order for Diazoxide (Hyperstat) is made. What should the nurse do during administration?

a. Use an infusion pump.

b. Place the client in Trendelenburg position.

c. Cover the solution with foil.

d. Assess the blood glucose level.

Answer D is correct. For hypertensive crisis, Hyperstat is given IV push. It frequently causes hyperglycemia. The glucose level will fall quickly following the administration of the medication. Answer A is incorrect because this medication is not administered via and infusion pump, but by IV push. Answer B is incorrect because the client must be placed in dorsal recumbent position. Answer C is incorrect because the drug is IV push.

48. Lanoxin elixir (digoxin) for the regulation of heart rate is being received by a six-month-old client with a ventricular septal defect. Which of the following findings should be reported to the doctor:

a. A blood pressure of 126/80

b. A heart rate of 60 bpm

c. A blood glucose of 110 mg/dl

d. A respiratory rate of 30 per minute

Answer B is correct. Bradycardia is linked with digoxin toxicity, therefore a heart rate of 60 in the six-month-old receiving Lanoxin elixir (digoxin) should be reported to the doctor immediately. Answers A, C, and D are incorrect because they are not linked with Lanozin administration.

49. A 55-year-old male with chest pain radiating to the jaw and left arm is admitted to the cardiac unit. In the diagnosis of a myocardial infarction, which enzyme would be most specific:

a. Aspartate aminotransferase

b. Lactic acid dehydrogenase

c. Creatine phosphokinase

d. Hydroxybutyric dehydrogenase

Answer C is correct. For a myocardial infarction, CK-MB (creatine phosphokinase muscle bond isoenzyme) is the most specific. Another one that is reliable is Troponin. Answers A, B, and D are incorrect because they are not specific to myocardial infarction.

50. A client is being taught about foods that are low in fat and cholesterol. Which of the following diet choices has the lowest levels of saturated fats?

a. Macaroni and cheese

b. Turkey breast

c. Shrimp with rice

d. Spaghetti and meatballs

Answer B is correct. Turkey contains the lowest amounts of fat and cholesterol. Answers A, C, and D are incorrect because a client on a low fat and cholesterol diet should avoid them.

51. A client is with left-sided congestive heart failure is admitted. What should the nurse check when assessing the client for edema?

a. Feet

b. Hands

c. Sacrum

d. Neck

Answer D is correct. In a client with congestive heart failure, the neck veins should be monitored for distension. Answers A and C are incorrect because Edema of the feet and hands are not an indication of central circulatory overload. Answer D is incorrect because Edema of the sacrum indicates right-sided congestive heart failure.

52. A client's central venous pressure is being checked by the nurse. Where should the nurse should place the zero of the manometer?

a. Point of maximum impulse (PMI)

b. Phlebostatic axis

c. Erb's point

d. Tail of Spence

Answer B is correct. The phlebostatic axis (at the fifth intercostal space mid-axillary line) is where the nurse should place the zero of the manometer when examining the central venous pressure. Answers A, C, and D are incorrect approaches.

53. Lisinopril (Zestril) and furosemide (Lasix) is ordered by the physician to be administered concomitantly to the client with hypertension. Which of the following should the nurse do:

a. Question the order.

b. Administer them separately.

c. Get it contact the pharmacy.

d. Administer the medications.

Answer D is correct. Zestril (an ACE inhibitor) is commonly given with a diuretics including Lasix. Answers A, B, and C are incorrect because it is unnecessary to question the order, administer the drugs individually, or get in contact the pharmacy.

54. What is the best process of evaluating the volume of peripheral edema?

a. Weighing the client daily

b. Measuring the intake and output

c. Measuring the extremity

d. Checking for pitting

Answer C is correct. Measuring the extremity the most effective method for evaluating the amount of peripheral edema. A paper tape measure should be used for an accurate assessment. Answers A, B, and D are incorrect because they are not the most effective methods for evaluating the amount of peripheral edema.

55. A low potassium diet is prescribed for a client with a renal failure. Which of the following food choices would be best for the client?

a. 1 cup beef broth

b. 1 cup rice

c. 1 baked potato with the skin

d. ½ cup raisins

Answer B is correct. A cup of rice is would be considered food that is low in potassium. Answers A, B, and D are incorrect because these foods contain greater amounts of potassium.

56. A client with an axillo-popliteal bypass graft is being prepared to discharge by the nurse. What should the client be instructed to avoid?

a. Sitting in a straight chair

b. The use of a recliner to rest

c. Resting in supine position

d. Sleep in right Sim's position

Answer A is correct. Activities that can obstruct the femoral artery graft should be avoided by a client with a axillo popliteal bypass graft. Because of this, sitting in a straight chair should be avoided. Answers B, C, and D are allowed, therefore they are incorrect answers.

57. Antithrombolic stockings have been ordered by the doctor to be placed on the legs of a client with peripheral vascular disease. How should the stockings be applied?

a. With the client in a standing position

b. Following bathing and applying powder

c. Prior to retiring in the evening

d. Prior to rising in the morning

Answer D is correct. In the morning before getting up is the optimal time to apply antithrombolytic stockings. If they are ordered for later in the day, the client should return to bed and wait for 30 minutes before applying them. Answers A, B, and C are incorrect because they will make the client more prone to be more peripheral edema.

59. The shift report has recently been received by the nurse who is getting prepared to make rounds. Which of the following clients should be seen first:

a. A client with a history of a cerebral aneurysm with an oxygen saturation rate of 99%

b. A client admitted one hour ago that has shortness of breath

c. A client three days post–coronary artery bypass graft with a temperature of 100.2°F

d. A client being prepared for discharge after a femoral popliteal bypass graft

Answer B is correct. A client that has recently been admitted with shortness of breath might need oxygen therapy and therefore should be seen first. Answer A is incorrect because the client is stable with an oxygen saturation rate of 99%. Answer C is incorrect because a temperature of 100.2°F is not uncommon due to the inflammatory process following surgery. Answer D is incorrect because the client can be attended to later because they are stable.

60. A client assigned to a partially private room with a femoral popliteal bypass graft. Who is the most suitable roommate for this client?

a. A client with diabetic ulcers

b. A client with ulcerative colitis

c. A client with hypothyroidism

d. A client with pneumonia

Answer C is correct. A client with hypothyroidism is the best roommate for the client after surgery. This is because the client is drowsy and is not infectious. Answers A, B, and D are incorrect because these clients could transmit infection to the client following a femoral popliteal bypass graft.

61. A client is being taught about the use sodium warfarin by the nurse. Which of the following statements by the

client would indicate that they require further instruction:

a. "My blood will be drawn every month."

b. "I will assess my skin for a rash."

c. "I will use an electric razor"

d. "I will take aspirin for a headache."

Answer D is correct. Taking aspirin while taking an anticoagulant will create additional bleeding, therefore they should not be taken. Answers A, B, and C are incorrect because they indicate a good understanding of sodium warfarin.

62. After repair of an abdominal aneurysm, a client returns to the recovery room. Which of the following findings would indicate a need to further investigation?

a. Pedal pulses regular

b. Blood pressure 108/50

c. Urinary output 20mL during the past hour

d. Oxygen saturation of 97%

Answer C is correct. The kidney's blood supply is impaired due to the the aorta being clamped throughout surgery. Renal damage can result from this. Oliguria is a urinary output of 20mL. Answer A is incorrect because the pedal pulses are within standard limits. Answer B is incorrect because it is appropriate that the client's blood pressure is slightly decreased after aneurysm surgical repair. Answer D is incorrect because the oxygen saturation is within normal range.

63. An order for heparin is made for a client who is admitted with thrombophlebitis. What should the medication be administered with?

a. A buretrol

b. An intravenous filter

c. An infusion controller

d. A three-way stop-cock

Answer C is correct. The nurse should utilize an infusion controller for the safe administering of heparin. If the infusion of heparin is too quick, this can result in hemorrhage. Answers A, B, and D are incorrect because they are unnecessary.

64. An obese client is having a blood pressure test. What will the results be if the blood pressure cuff is too small?

a. A reading that is falsely low

b. A reading that is falsely elevated

c. A blood pressure reading that is correct

d. A subnormal finding

Answer B is correct. When a blood pressure cuff is too small, this will result in a blood pressure that is falsely elevated. Answers A, C, and D are incorrect.

65. Preparation for surgery is occurring for a client with an abdominal aortic aneurysm. What should be reported to the doctor?

a. An abdominal bruit

b. A negative Babinski reflex

c. An elevation of white blood cell count

d. Pupils that are equal and reactive to light

Answer C is correct. An elevated white blood cell count indicated an infection and therefore should be reported to the doctor. Answers A, B, and D are incorrect because they are expected.

66. A client's pulmonary artery pressure is being evaluated by the nurse. Which of the following does this test evaluate?

a. The systolic, diastolic, and mean pressure of the pulmonary artery

b. The left ventricle pressure

c. The pulmonary veins pressure

d. The right ventricle pressure

Answer A is correct. Pressure during systole, diastole, and the mean pulmonary artery pressure will be measured by the pulmonary artery pressure. Answers B, C, are incorrect because they will not be measured.

67. A central venous pressure monitor is being used to monitor a client. What should the nurse do if the pressure is .5cm of water?

a. Inform the doctor immediately

b. Slow down the intravenous infusion

c. Listen to the lungs for rales

d. Administer a diuretic

Answer A is correct. A.5cm pressure is low and the doctor should be informed of this immediately. Answers B, C, and D would indicate that the reading is too high and therefore they are incorrect.

68. Ventricular tachycardia on the heart monitor is identified by the nurse. The client has a pulse. What should the nurse immediately do?

a. Administer atropine sulfate

b. Prepare to administer an antiarrhythmic medication

c. Check the level of potassium

d. Defibrillate at 360 joules

Answer B is correct. A medication that will slow down and correct the abnormal rhythm is the required treatment for ventricular tachycardia. Answer A is incorrect because atropine sulfate will increase the rate further. Answer C is incorrect because checking the potassium is not a priority. Answer D is incorrect because defibrillation is only utilized for pulseless ventricular tachycardia/ventricular fibrillation (*Remember: defibrillation would start at 200 joules, increasing to 360 joules*).

69. If a client is taking warfarin sodium (Coumadin), which of the following lab studies should be done regularly?

a. White blood cell count

b. Blood glucose

c. Erthyrocyte count

d. Stool specimen for occult blood

Answer D is correct. In order to detect any intestinal bleeding on the client with Coumadin therapy, an occult blood test should be done regularly. Answers A, B, and C are not entirely relevant to the question.

70. To prevent post-surgical thrombi, a client has an order for heparin. What should the nurse do immediately following the heparin injection?

a. Check the site for bleeding

b. Aspirate for blood

c. Check the pulse rate

d. Massage the site

Answer A is correct. The nurse should check the site for bleeding after administering any subcutaneous anticoagulant. Answers B and D are incorrect because these are incorrect actions. Answer C is incorrect because checking the pulse in unnecessary.

71. The client is admitted to the emergency room. They have anxiety, shortness of breath, and tachycardia. Their ECG shows atrial fibrillation, along with a ventricular response rate of 130 beats per minute. An order for quinidine sulfate is made by the doctor. What should the nurse monitor the client's ECG for while they are receiving quinidine?

a. Peaked P wave

b. Elevated ST segment

c. Prolonged QT interval

d. Inverted T wave

Answer C is correct. Widened QT intervals and heart block can be cause by quinidine. Notched P waves and widened QRS complexes are some other signs of myocardial toxicity. Answers A, B, and D are not relevant to quinidine use.

72. A client with thrombophlebitis of the left lower extremity is receiving heparin. Which drug reverses the effects of heparin?

a. Protamine sulfate

b. Cyanocobalamine

c. Streptokinase

d. Sodium warfarin

Answer A is correct. Protamine sulfate the antidote for heparin. Answers B, C , and D are anticoagulants therefore they are incorrect.

73. A client has returned to the unit from surgery. They have a blood pressure of 90/50, pulse 132, and respirations 30. Which of the following actions should receive priority from the nurse?

a. Continue to monitor the vital signs

b. Ask the client how he feels

c. Contact the physician

d. Ask the LPN to continue the post-op care

Answer C is correct. This should be reported to the doctor immediately because the vital signs are abnormal. Answer A is incorrect because continuing to monitor the signs can create a further deterioration in the client's conditions. Answer B is incorrect because this would provide only subjective data. Answer D is incorrect because getting the LPN involved is not the optimal solution.

74. Sodium warfarin is ordered by the physician for a client with thrombophlebitis. What time should the medication be administered at?

a. 09.00

b. 12.00

c. 17.00

d. 21.00

Answer C is correct. Sodium warfarin should be administered in the late afternoon, at approx. 17.00 hours. This allows for correct bleeding times to be taken in the morning. A, B, and D are incorrect.

75. What should the nurse do to ensure safety while administering a nitroglycerine patch?

a. Shave the area where the patch will be applied.

b. Wear gloves while applying the patch.

c. Wash the area with soap and rinse with hot water.

d. Apply the patch to the buttocks.

Answer B is correct. To protect himself or herself, the nurse should wear gloves when applying a nitroglycerine patch/cream. Answer A is incorrect because shaving the shin could graze the area. Washing the area with hot water will vasodilate and increase absorption, therefore answer C is incorrect. Answer D is incorrect because the patches should be applied to an area that is above the waist.

76. **The nurse is caring for a female client with a myocardial infarction. The client enters the nurse's station informing the nurses that she is ready to be discharged because there is nothing wrong with her. Which of the following defense mechanism is the client employing?**

a. Conversion reaction

b. Denial

c. Projection

d. Rationalization

Answer B is correct. The client who states that there is nothing wrong with them is in a state denial. Answer A is incorrect because conversion reaction is when a client converts a psychological trauma into a physical illness. Answer C is incorrect because projection is the action of projecting thoughts or feeling onto others. Answer D is also incorrect because rationalization is the act of making excuses for what happened.

77. The graduate nurse is recording the central venous pressure. Which of the following observations would indicate to the nurse that the graduate requires further teaching?

a. The graduate nurse is turning the stop-cock to the off position from the IV fluid to the client.

b. The graduate nurse is teaching the client to perform the Valsalva maneuver during the CVP reading.

c. The graduate nurse is positioning the client in a supine position in order to read the manometer.

d. The graduate nurse is noting the level at the top of the meniscus.

Answer B is correct. If the graduate nurse instructs the client to perform the Valsalva maneuver, this is an indication that the graduate nurse requires further teaching. This is because clients should not be instructed to do the Valsalva maneuver during central venous pressure readings. Answers A, C, and D are all incorrect because these are all correct ways in which to assess central venous pressure.

78. The nurse has been assigned to a client who has been scheduled for a surgical repair of a saccular abdominal aortic aneurysm. Which of the following pre-op assessments should the nurse prioritize?

a. Assessment of bowel sounds and activity

b. Assessment of the client's anxiety levels

c. Evaluation of the client's exercise tolerance

d. Identification of peripheral pulses

Answer D is correct. During the surgery, the aorta is clamped. Because of this, the nurse should prioritize the identification of peripheral pulses during the preoperative period. On top of this, the nurse should also assess the return of circulation to the lower extremities.

Answer B is incorrect because it is of little concern in the preoperative period. And answer A is incorrect because it is of even lesser concern at this time. Answer C is incorrect because evaluating the client's exercise tolerance does not need to be assessed at this moment in time.

79. The nurse is preparing a client with an implantable defibrillator for discharge. Which of the following should the nurse include on the client's teaching plan?

a. "You will not be able to fly in an airplane with the defibrillator in place."

b. "You should only use your cell phone on your right side."

c. "You cannot eat microwave food."

d. "Avoid moving the shoulder on the side of the pacemaker site for six weeks."

Answer B is correct. The nurse should instruct the client with an internal defibrillator to only use their cell phone as well as any other battery-operated devices on the opposite site. On top of this, the nurse should also advise the client to immediately report dizziness and fainting and teach the client to take their pulse rate. Answers A, C, and D are all incorrect because they are incorrect statements.

80. The nurse is caring for a male client who is experiencing fetal heart rates of 100–110 beats per minute during the contractions. Which of the following actions should the nurse prioritize?

a. Apply an internal monitorA

b. Assist the client to get up and walk him in the hallC

c. Move the client to the delivery roomD

d. Turn the client to his left side

Answer D is correct. The nurse should prioritize turning the client to his left side and supplying oxygen. The normal fetal heart rate ranges from 120–160bpm. A heart rate of 100–110bpm therefore indicates that the client is experiencing bradycardia. Answer A is incorrect because it is not applicable at this time. Answer B is incorrect because this is not a good action for a client with bradycardia. Answer C is also incorrect because moving the client to the delivery room is not a good action to take given the situation.

81. Which of the following findings is indicative of a reassuring fetal heart rate pattern?

a. Acceleration of FHR with fetal movements

b. A fetal heart rate of 90 at the baseline

c .A fetal heart rate of 180bpm

d. A baseline variability of 35bpm

Answer A is correct. This is because accelerations of FHR with fetal movement are normal and is therefore a reassuring fetal heart rate pattern. Answer B, C, and D are all incorrect because these are not reassuring fetal heart rate patterns.

82. The nurse is caring for a client with congestive heart failure has been maintained on digoxin (Lanoxin). Which of the following findings indicates to the nurse that the drug is having its intended effect?

a. Improved appetite

b. Increased pedal edema

c. Increased urinary output

d. Stabilized weight

Answer C is correct. An increase in the client's urinary output is indicative of the fact that the drug is having its desired effect of eliminating excess fluid from the client's body. This is because the effect of Lanoxin is to slow and strengthen the contraction of the heart. Answer A is incorrect because improved appetite is not an effect that is associated to the drug. Answer B is incorrect because pedal edema would decrease, not increase. Answer D is also incorrect because the client's weight would decrease, and not remain stable.

83. The client with suspected abdominal aortic aneurysm (AAA) is admitted ot the hospital. Which of the following can the nurse expect the client with an abdominal aortic aneurysm to experience?

a. A decrease in urinary output

b. A loss of sensation in the lower extremities

c. Back pain that is slightly diminished when standing

d. Pulsations in the periumbilical area

Answer D is correct. It is common for clients with an abdominal aortic aneurysm to experience feeling the heart beat in the in the abdomen. Answer A and B are incorrect because these are not related to abdominal aortic aneurysm. Answer C is also incorrect because back pain is not impacted by changes in position.

84. The nurse has been assigned to a three-year-old year old client with a diagnosis of Kawasaki's disease. Which of the following is a severe complication that can arise in clients with Kawasaki's disease?

a. The development of a giant aneurysm

b. The development of Brushfield spots

c. The development of coxa plana

d. The eruption of Hutchinson's teeth

Answer A is correct. The development of a giant aneurysm is a severe complication that can arise in clients with Kawasaki's disease. Answers B, C, and D are all incorrect because these are not associated with the disease.

85. The nurse is caring for client with an order for Coumadin (sodium warfarin) who is experiencing transient ischemic attacks. Which of the following findings measures the therapeutic level of Coumadin?

a. Bleeding time

b. Clot retraction time

c. Partial thromboplastin time

d. Prothrombin time

Answer D is correct. This is because the therapeutic level of Coumadin is measured by the prothrombin time. Answer A is incorrect because bleeding time measures the vascular and platelet factors that are associated with hemostasis. Answer B is incorrect because clot retraction time is a measure to assess the quantity of each specific clotting factor. Answer C is also incorrect because partial thromboplastin time is used to measure the the therapeutic level of heparin, and not of Coumadin.

86. The client with a myocardial infarction has been admitted to the unit. Which of the following is the most common complication that arises in clients after a myocardial infarction?

a. Cardiac dysrhythmia

b. Hyperkalemia

c. Left ventricular hypertrophy

d. Right ventricular hypertrophy

Answer A is correct. This is because clients with a myocardial infarction are at most risk of developing cardiac dysrhythmias. Answer B is incorrect because hyperkalemia is not the most common complication that arises after a myocardial infarction. Answer C and D are also incorrect because these are not associated with myocardial infarctions.

87. The nurse is caring for a client who has just undergone a coronary artery bypass surgery. The nurse notices that the client has developed a temperature of 102°F. The nurse knows to immediately notify the doctor because elevations in the client's temperature causes which of the following?

a. A decreased cardiac output

b. An increased cardiac output

c. Cardiac tamponade

d. Graft rejection

Answer B is correct. The nurse should immediately notify the doctor because an increase in temperature increases the cardiac output. Answer A is incorrect because an increase in temperature does not decrease the cardiac output. Answer C is incorrect because cardiac tamponade has no relationship to elevations in temperature. Answer D is also incorrect because clients with a coronary artery bypass graft and an elevated temperature are most likely experiencing inflammation and not a graft rejection.

88. The nurse has been assigned to a client who has just undergone coronary artery bypass graft (CABG). When performing a nursing, the nurse should prioritize reporting which of the following findings?

a. Urinary output of 40mL per hour

b. Restlessness and confusion

c. Pallor and coolness of skin

d. Chest drainage of 150mL in the past hour

Answer D is correct. The nurse should immediately notify the doctor of the client's chest drainage because a chest drainage which is greater than 100mL per hour is excessive and indicative of a potential hemorrhage. Answer A is incorrect because the urinary output given is within its normal range. Answer B is incorrect because these symptoms could be a response to the client experiencing pain, oxygen changes, or another factor. Answer C is also incorrect because this is an expected side effect in clients who have just undergone a CABG.

89. The nurse is caring for a client who has an order of of Lanoxin (digoxin) to be administered in the morning. When checking the apical pulse rate however, the nurse notes a rate of 54. Which of the following is the appropriate nursing action?

a. Withhold the medication until the client's heart rate increases

b. Withhold the medication and notify the physician

c. Record the pulse rate and administer the medication as usual

d. Administer the medication and monitor the client's heart rate

Answer B is correct. The correct intervention for the

nurse to take is to withhold the medication and to notify the physician. Answers A, C, and D are all incorrect because these nursing actions do not provide for the safety of the client.

90. The home health nurse is visiting a client with congestive heart failure who has been maintained. Which of the following medications puts the client at risk of developing hypokalemia?

a. Midamor (amiloride hydrochloride)

b. Dyrenium (triamterene)

c. Demadex (torsemide)

d. Aldactone (spironolactone)

Answer C is correct. This is because the medication Demadex is a loop diuretic that depletes potassium. Answers A, B, and D are incorrect because Midamor, Dyrenium, and Aldactone are all potassium-sparing diuretics.

The nurse is caring for a client with stable angina who has an order for nitroglycerin buccal tablets. The nurse is aware that nitroglycerin causes which of the following?

a. A decrease in the rate of contractions of the heart

b. An increase in the ventricular fill time

c. It dilates coronary blood vessels

d. It strengthens the contractions of the heart

Answer C is correct. The nurse knows that the effect of Nitroglycerin is to dilate coronary blood vessels, thereby improving circulation to the myocardium. Answers A, B, and D are all incorrect because they all describe the effects of the medication Digoxin.

92. Which of the following is a suitable activity for a client who has suffered an uncomplicated myocardial infarction (MI) less than 48 hours ago?

a. Ambulating in the room and hall as tolerated

b. Remaining on strict bed rest with bedside commode privileges

c. Sitting on the bedside for five minutes three times a day with assistance

d. Sitting upright in the bedside chair for 15 minutes two to three times every day

Answer C is correct. Clients who have recently experienced an MI should only be allowed to sit on the side of the bed for five minutes three times a day. Assistance should always be provided. Answer A and D are both incorrect because they would increase the workload on the heart too much and too soon. Answer B is also incorrect because the client should be allowed some activity.

93. The nurse has been instructing the client with hypertension on the role of diet in regulating blood pressure. Which of the following food choices would indicate to the nurse that the client has understood the teachings?

a. Cornflakes, banana, milk, and coffee

b. Dry toast, oatmeal, apple juice, and coffee

c. Pancakes, tomato juice, ham, and tea

d. Scrambled eggs, toast, bacon, and coffee

Answer B is correct. This is because oatmeal is both high in fiber and low in sodium. Clients with hypertension should be encouraged to strictly adopt a diet that is low in sodium, high-fiber and low-cholesterol. Answer A is incorrect because this meal choice is high in sodium and low in fiber. Answer C and D are also incorrect because they both animal proteins which are high in cholesterol and high in sodium.

94. Which of the following is a common finding in clients with right-sided heart failure?

a. Crackles in the lungs

b. Daytime oliguria

c. Nocturnal polyuria

d. Shortness of breath

Answer C is correct. Clients with right-sided heart failure are likely to experience increased voiding during the night. Answers A, B, and D are all incorrect because these are all symptoms associated with left-sided heart failure.

95. The nurse is caring for a client with anemia. Which of the following findings would be most indicative of the anemia?

a. BP 146/88

b. Pink complexion

c. Respirations 28 shallow

d. Weight gain of 12 pounds in six months

Answer C is correct. Clients with anemia are often short of breath. This is because a decrease in red blood cells results in less oxygen and less hemoglobin. Answer A is incorrect because clients with anemia are likely to experience hypotension. Answer B is also incorrect because the client with anemia will appear pale. Answer D is also incorrect because clients with anemia will experience weight loss, and not weight gain.

96. The nurse is caring for a six-month-old client with a ventral septal defect who has been maintained Digitalis. The medication has been prescribed in order to regulate her heart rate. Which of the following findings should the nurse immediately reported to the doctor?

a. Respiratory rate of 30 per minute

b. Heart rate of 60bpm

c. Blood pressure of 126/80

d. Blood glucose of 110mg/dL

Answer B is correct. The nurse should immediately report a heart rate of 60. The medication should be withheld if the heart rate is below 100bpm. Answers A, C, and D are all incorrect because the values given are all within their normal range.

97. The physician has ordered nitroglycerine for the client with angina. Which of the following instructions should the nurse give to the client?

a. "Replenish your supply every three months."

b. "Take one pill every 15 minutes if you experience pain."

c. "Leave the medication in the brown bottle."

d. "Crush the medication and swallow with water."

Answer C is correct. The nurse should instruct the client to keep the medication in the brown bottle. This is because Nitroglycerine is instable and tends to become less potent if exposed to light, air, or water. Answer A is incorrect because the medication should be replenished every six months. Answer B is incorrect because the client should be instructed to take one tablet every five minutes until pain subsides. Answer D is also incorrect because the medication should not be crushed.

98. The doctor has instructed the client to be placed on a low-fat and low-cholesterol diet. Which of the following meal choices contains the lowest amount of

saturated fats?

a. Macaroni and cheese

b. Shrimp with rice

c. Spaghetti with meat sauce

d. Turkey breast

Answer D is correct. This is because turkey contains the lowest amount of cholesterol and fats. The client should also be taught to bake the meat rather than to fry it in order to keep the fat content as low as possible. Answers A, B, and C are all incorrect because the client should be instructed to avoid foods such as beef, cheese, chocolate, cream sauces, eggs, liver, and shrimp.

99. The client with left-sided congestive heart failure is admitted to the unit. Which of the following should the nurse check when assessing the client for edema?

a. Feet

b. Hands

c. Neck

d. Sacrum

Answer C is correct. The nurse should assess the client's neck because the jugular veins in the neck should be checked for distension. Answer A, B, and D are all incorrect because checking these body parts will be edematous in right-sided congestive heart failure.

100. When assessing a client's central venous pressure, which of the following should the zero of the manometer be placed at?

a. The Erb's point

b. The phlebostatic axis

c. The point of maximal impulse (PMI)

d. The Tail of Spence (the upper outer quadrant of the breast)

Answer B is correct. This is because the phlebostatic axis is the correct placement for the manometer. The axis can be found l at the fifth intercostals space midaxillary line. Answer C is incorrect because the Erb's point where the nurse can hear the valves close simultaneously. Answer C is incorrect because the PMI is located at the fifth intercostals space midclavicular line. Answer D is also incorrect because the Tail of Spence has no relation with the placement of a manometer and is therefore entirely unrelated.

101. The physician has ordered Protime of 120 seconds for a client with sodium warfarin (Coumadin). Which of the following nursing interventions is of most importance at this time?

a. Anticipating an increase in the Coumadin dosage

b. Assessment for signs of abnormal bleeding

c. Increasing the frequency of neurological assessments

d. Teaching the client about the drug therapy

Answer B is correct. The nurse should prioritize assessing the client for signs of abnormal bleeding. This is because a Protime of 120 seconds indicates an extremely prolonged Protime (normal Protime is roughly 12–20 seconds), which can result in spontaneous bleeding. Answers A, C, and D are all incorrect because they are not a priority at this time and can be taken at a later time.

102. The nurse his caring for a client who has been admitted to the emergency room. The client suffers from substernal chest pain that is radiating to the left jaw. Which of the following ECG findings indicates to the nurse that the client may be experiencing acute myocardial infarction?

a. Changes in ST segment

b. Minimal QRS wave

c. Peaked P wave

d. Prominent U wave

Answer A is correct. This is because changes in the ST segment are indicative of acute myocardial infraction. Answers B, C, and D are all incorrect because minimal QRS waves, peaked P waves, and prominent U waves are not indications of acute myocardial infarction.

The Respiratory System

Section 1: Introduction to the Respiratory System

Lung disease is the third leading cause of death for people aged 55-65 years old in America (Centers for Disease Control, 2010). According to estimations, over 35 million people in the United States are affected by chronic lung disease. A number of these lung diseases are due to occupational exposure and produce risks of lung cancer. On top of this, respiratory infections are the cause of many infections acquired in the hospital.

It is important to spend enough time reviewing the care of clients with respiratory disorders in your preparation for the NCLEX. On top of this, it is also crucial to practice applying your knowledge with multiple practice questions. This concise preparation guide will cover the key points that you will need to know to be successful in the respiratory portion of your NCLEX test.

The guide begins with an outline of the topics and key facts on respiratory disorders that you need to remember for the exam. The list of subtopics can be seen on the contents page. In Section 7 of this guide you can apply and test your knowledge with over 100 topic-specific practice questions. All answers to the questions are given, along with detailed rationales to further your knowledge and understanding of the topic.

Remember that ambition is the first step to success. The second step is action – hard work and determination. Purchasing this guide is an indication of your ambition, now it's time to get to work!

Best wishes,

Eva Regan

Section 2: Lower Respiratory Tract Noninfectious Disorders

The exchange of oxygen and carbon dioxide are affected by noninfectious disorders of the lower respiratory tract. Some of these noninfectious disorders are preventable and some are not. This section covers the key points you need to know for each type.

<u>Chronic Bronchitis</u>

Key points
- An inflammation of the bronchioles and bronchi.
- Caused by ongoing exposure to infections or noninfectious irritants (e.g. smoke from tobacco)
- Bronchitis is limited to the small and large airways.
- Bronchial wall thickening and mucus congests small airways and makes large airways narrower.
- The removal of irritants can often reverse chronic bronchitis.
- Respiratory infections can lead chronic bronchitis to develop to right-sided heart failure, pulmonary hypertension, and sometimes acute respiratory failure.
- Most common in 40 - 55 years old.

Symptoms
- Shortness of breath
- Coughing
- Coughing which masters 3 months+ for 2 years
- Sputum production
- Eating difficulties
- Weight loss
- Difficulty sleeping

• Crackles and wheezes

Treatment
• Bronchodilators
• Steroids
• Antacid.
• Expectorants
• Antibiotics (if acute respiratory infection)
• Correcting imbalances in acid/base
• Improving nutritional requirements
• Regular oral care
• Providing oxygen (low settings)

Emphysema

Key Points
• Alveoli overdistention (irreversible).
• Alveolar wall destruction.
• Clients can be described as 'pink puffers' - involves bronchiole, alveolar duct, and alveoli. They experience exertion dyspnea and remain pink.
• Clients can also be described as 'blue bloaters' - involves secondary lobule, produces changes in oxygen perfusion. They experience chronic hypoxia, cyanosis, pulmonary edema (occasionally respiratory failure). Also experience dyspnea and cyanosis.
• Can lead to development of clots due to polycythemia.

Symptoms
• Barrel chest
• Digital clubbing
• Shallow respirations (shallow)
• Expiratory phase, grunting respirations
• Muscle atrophy
• Weight loss

- Cyanosis (peripheral)
- Forceful coughing of sputum

- The flattening of the diaphragm will be seen from a chest x-ray.
- Increased carbon dioxide and decreased oxygen levels are shown in arterial blood gases.
- Increased residual volume and decreased vital capacity.
- a1-antitrypsin levels can be observed for lack of the enzyme
- normal levels range from 80 - 260 mg/dL.

Many symptoms of emphysema are similar to those of chronic bronchitis.

Treatment
- Bronchodilators (can be administered by dose inhaler, dry powder inhaler, orally, nebulizer)
- Steroids
- Antacids
- Expectorants
- Antibiotics (if acute respiratory infection)
- Bronchodilators administrated orally have more adverse effects.
- Prophylactic antibiotics might be used for those with 4+ yearly respiratory infections.
- Pneumococcal pneumonia immunization and influenza vaccinations yearly are recommended - reduces respiratory infection risks.
- Acid/base imbalance corrections.
- Improving nutritional requirements.
- Regular oral care.
- Providing oxygen (low settings).

Asthma

Key points
- Common childhood respiratory condition.
- *Intrinsic asthma* - Cold temperature exposure or infection.
- *Extrinsic asthma* - Frequently linked with eczema in childhood.
- Asthma and eczema can both be triggered by food allergies.
- Gradual introduction to new foods for children reduces allergies.
- Asthma can occur at any age.

Symptoms
- Wheezing
- Breath shortness
- Dry cough
- Thick and white sputum
- Severe asthma attack can result in asthmaticus - possible respiratory collapse/death

Treatment
- Maintenance therapy - mast cell stabilizers, leukotriene modifiers.
- Acute asthma attacks can be treated with oral/inhaled B2 agonists, along with anti-inflammatories. For example, short acting: Albuterolter and butaline, long acting: salmetrol.

It is important for the nurse to instruct the client of the correct use of a metered-dose and dry-powder inhaler.

Use of Metered-Dose Inhaler:
1. Insert inhaler canister into mouthpiece.
2. Remove cap of mouthpiece, shake canister for 5 seconds.
3. Slow and deep exhale.
4. Hold canister upside down and 1-2 inches away from the mouth.

5. Deep inhale for 3 to 5 seconds, pressing down on canister
6. Hold breath (10 seconds), release canister, then slow exhalation.
7. Wait 1 minute before carrying out the procedure again
8. Rinse mouthpiece/spacer and place in sterile area.

Dry-Powder Inhaler:
Should be stored in a dry area.

1. Hold inhaler upright and remove cap.
2. Load inhaler.
3. Hold inhaler in line with mouthpiece.
4. Slight tilt of the head backwards
5. Insert mouthpiece into mouth, seal with lips.
6. Deep inhale for 3 seconds
7. Hold breath (10 seconds), remove inhaler
8. Slow exhalation
9. Rinse mouth, brush teeth
10. Store inhaler in sterile are in sealed bag

Pleurisy (Pleuritis)

Key Points
• Pleural sac inflammation
• Possibly linked with respiratory infection (upper), pulmonary embolus, cancer, thoracotomy, and chest trauma.

Symptoms
• Inspiration pain
• Fever
• Chills
• Dyspnea
• Cough
• Air or fluid in pleural sac seen in chest x-ray.

Treatment
• Analgesics administration (Indocin, NSAIDS)
• Antitussives with codeine
• Antibiotics
• Oxygen therapy
• Thoracentesis for pleural effusion

For thoracentesis, the nurse should prepare the client by putting them in the correct positioning:

• Sitting on edge of a bed with arms and head placed on an over the bed table (padded).
• Sitting on a chair with head and arms resting on back of chair.

Pulmonary Hypertension

Key Points
• Vascular resistance in the lungs due to constriction of blood vessels.
• Systolic pressures larger than 30mm Hg in pulmonary artery.
• Can be caused due to other lung disorders.
• Primary pulmonary hypertension has an unknown cause.
• 50% of affected with familial have a bone mutation - results in morphogenetic protein receptor. They have 10% to 20% chance of generating pulmonary hypertension.
• Common in families and females aged 20-40.

Symptoms
• Chest pain
• Dyspnea
• Fatigue
• Eventual failure of right side of the heart

Diagnosis:
- Right side heart catheterization - shows increased pressure in the pulmonary artery.
- Decreased pulmonary volumes, decreased diffusion capacity.
- Confirmation of diagnosis via abnormal ventilation perfusion scan, abnormal spiral CT.

Treatment
- Anticoagulants
- Cardiotonics
- Vasodilators
- Bronchodilators
- Calcium channel blockers
- Diuretics
- Daily doses of Coumadin/Warfarin - to reach 1.5 to 2.0 international normalized ratio. (Can prevent thrombosis).
- Cardizem and calcium channel blockers (e.g. Pericardia) to dilate blood vessels.
- Short acting direct vasodilators (e.g. Flolan, Remodulin, Tracleer).
- Limited use of vasodilators - they can produce systemic hypotension.
- Infusion of adenosine into the pulmonary artery.

Interstitial Pulmonary (Fibrotic Lung) Disease

Key Points
- Includes a number of lung diseases.
- Pathologic changes in the blood vessels, alveoli, and lung support tissues.
- Thickening of lung tissue - 'stiff' lung.
- Restriction in expansion.

Examples: Idiopathic pulmonary fibrosis and Sarcoidosis

Sarcoidosis

Key Points
- Can produce granulomatous lesions in most organs and tissues.
- Hypersensitive response to bacteria, fungi, chemicals, viruses.
- Lungs, spleen, lymph nodes, central nervous system, liver, eyes, and skin are usually affected.
- Granulomatous infiltration and fibrosis create low lung compliance.

Symptoms
- Dyspnea
- Hemoptysis
- Congestion
- Fatigue
- Weight loss
- Fever

Diagnosis: CT scan and chest x-ray - disseminated miliary, lesions in the lungs.

Treatment
- Clients sometimes see remission with no treatment.
- Cytotoxic or immunosuppressive medication.
- Corticosteroids
- Plaquenil
- Indocin
- Imuran
- Rheumatrex

Pulmonary Fibrosis

Key Points
- Common in older cigarette smokers, or exposure to metal particles and organic chemicals.
- Injured lungs create process of inflammation.
- Damaged alveoli.
- Clients generally have worsening symptoms.
- Despite treatment, most die within 5 years.

Symptoms
- Mild exertional dyspnea.
- Severe dyspnea and hypoxemia.

Treatment
- Immunosuppressive drugs: Cytoxan, Imuran - to reduce inflammation
- Curative lung transplant.

Occupational Pulmonary Disease

Key Points
- Caused by exposure to organic / inorganic dusts, noxious fumes in the workplace.
- Other pulmonary irritants (e.g. cigarette smoke) increase the risk of lung cancer.
- Examples of occupational pulmonary diseases: pneumoconiosis, asbestosis, silicosis, talcosis, berylliosis.

Adequate ventilation of the workplace and protective equipment prevents occupational pulmonary disease.

Section 3: Lower Respiratory Tract Infectious Disorders

Infectious disorders of the lower respiratory tract are diseases that affect the lung.

Pneumonia

Key Points
- Inflammation of the parenchyma - caused by bacteria, viruses and fungi.
- **Community acquired:** Treptococcal pneumonia, Legionnaires' disease, Haemophilus influenza, Mycoplasma pneumoniae, viral pneumonia, chlamydial pneumonia.
- **Hospital acquired:** Pseudomonas pneumonia, staphylococcal pneumonia, Pneumocystis carinii pneumonia (PCP), Klebsiella pneumonia, fungal pneumonia.

Symptoms
- Hypoxia
- Tachycardia
- Tachypnea
- Malaise
- Fever

Viral pneumonia symptoms are generally milder.

Treatment
Bacterial pneumonia:
- Antibiotics
- Antipyretics
- Antitussives

- Oxygen
- Meeteing nutritional needs.
- Improving oral hygiene.

Viral pneumonia is treated with antiviral therapy, and fungal pneumonia with antifungal therapy.

The pneumococcal vaccine generally gives lifelong immunity, and is recommended for those aged 65+ and cardiorespiratory conditions.

Oxygen Therapy

- Reduces workload of lungs and heart by providing oxygen to the blood. Oxygen systems are 'low flow' or 'high flow':

Low flow: e.g. Nasal cannulas, masks. Give oxygen while the clients continues to breath.

High flow: Venturi, aerosol masks.

Nurses should watch for signs of oxygen toxicity: paresthesias, dyspnea, restlessness, malaise, and fatigue.

Chest Physiotherapy

- Percussion, vibration and drainage to remove bronchial secretions.
- Improves oxygenation.
- Should not be carried out on clients that have had thoracic surgery recently.

Process: Rhythmic strikes of the chest with cupped hands for up to 5 minutes on each lung area.

Tuberculosis

Key Points
- Respiratory infection.
- Caused by mycobacterium tuberculosis.
- Contagious.
- Risk factors: overcrowded living, age, and immune compromise.

Symptoms
- Some may show no symptoms
- Fever
- Loss of weight
- Indigestion
- Coughing
- Night sweats
- Breath shortness

The kidney, spine, lungs, and cervical lymph nodes are usually affected by tuberculosis.

Testing
- Intradermal PPD test:
- Injecting 0.1ml of PPd in the inner aspect of the forearm.
- Reading taken in 48 to 72 hours.
0-4mm induration = generally negative.
5-9mm induration = questionable exposure.
5-9mm induration = positive for those immunocompromised, with HIV, and abnormal chest x-ray.
10-14mm induration = positive for those born in TB prevalent country, drug users, with malnutrition and diabetes.
15+ indurations = generally considered positive for all.

A positive result does not mean an active disease - clients should have an x-ray to detect active tuberculosis.

Tuberculosis is confirmed by a sputum test.

Treatment
- Antimycobacterial drugs INH (isoniazid)
- Myambutol
- Rifadin
- Streptomycin
- Tebrazid

- Combined medication reduces treatment time which is generally 6 months. HIV positive clients generally require treatment for 9 months.
- Other members of the client's household should be checked for tuberculosis.
- Sputum specimens are taken every 2 to 4 weeks - 3 negative sputum tests allow the client to return to work.

Influenza

Key Points
- Viral infection of upper respiratory tract.
- Highly contagious.
- Caused by Myxovirus influenzae.
- Immunization is required annually.

Symptoms
- Chills
- Laryngistis
- Sore throat
- Muscle aches
- Runny nose
- Fever (Over 102 degrees)

Influenza can cause pneumonia and myositis, pericarditis, encephalitis.

Prevention:
- Vaccine should be given to the elderly, children, and clients with chronic illness.
- Vaccine is given in the fall.

Treatment
- Rest and adequate fluid intake.
- Nasal sprays.
- Antitussives with codeine.
- Antipyretics.
- Antibiotics (if client has bacterial pneumonia).
- Antivirals: Relenza and Tamiflu.
- Symmetrel.
- Flumadine.

Section 4: Life-Threatening Pulmonary Disorders

Respiratory disorders can quickly progress into stages where life saving measures need to be taken. Here are the common life threatening respiratory disorders, along with their care processes.

Acute Respiratory Distress Syndrome (ARDS)

Key Points
- Generally occurs in those that are otherwise healthy.
- Caused by intrinsic factors: e.g. anaphylaxis, pulmonary emboli, or extrinsic factors: e.g. inhalation injury.
- Extravascular lung fluid, interstitial tissue remains dry.

Diagnosis:
- Chest x-ray that shows emphysematous changes
- Lungs have 'ground glass' appearance.
- Hypoxia.
- Crackles.
- Refractory hypoxemia (low blood oxygen levels).

Nursing Care:
- Continuous Positive Airway Pressure (CPAP)
- Endotrachial intubation and mechanical ventilation with positive end expiratory pressure (PEEP)
- Arterial blood gas monitoring.
- Meeting nutritional needs (e.g. tube feeding)
- Maintain cardiac output tissue perfusion.
- Pulmonary artery wedge pressure monitoring.
- Changes in the client's position.
- Sepsis, pneumonia, and multi-system organ dysfunction prevention.

• Preventing thrombophlebitis by using low molecular weight heparin.

Mechanical Ventilation
ARDS presents problems with maintaining gas exchange - mechanical ventilation is generally necessary.

Types of ventilators:
Negative-pressure ventilators - Involves chest cavity pressure changes e.g. the body wrap or poncho. Artificial airways are unnecessary.

Positive-pressure ventilators - Lungs are inflated via positive pressure on the airway. Expansion of alveoli. A tracheostomy or endotracheal tube are generally needed. They have different classifications:
- Pressure-cycled ventilators: A preset airway pressure is gained by pushing air into the lungs. Generally used for respiratory therapy.
- Volume-cycled ventilators: A preset volume is delivered by pushing air into to the lungs. Determined pressure limits excessive pressure.
- Time-cycled ventilators: Air pushed into lungs for a set period of time.

Controlling modes of ventilators:

Controlled - Set tidal volume and respiratory rate determines the ventilation of the machine. Any spontaneous respirations are prevented.

Assist controlled - Set oxygen volume is given at a set rate. Negative inspiratory effort from the client can prompt ventilations.

Synchronized intermittent mandatory - Set number of respirations given. Spontaneous breaths can be taken.

Guidelines for settings on ventilator:
• Tidal volume should be set 10 to 15 mL/Kg.
• Lowest concentration of oxygen should be set to maintain aO2 of 80 to 100 mm Hg.
• Set mode.
• Ensure client can trigger the ventilator easy by adjusting the sensitivity.
• Take record of minute volume, measurement of Pa02, PaCO2, and pH in 20 minute intervals.
• Adjustment of settings based on arterial blood gas, maintain prescribed levels.
• Make assessments for hypoxemia if confusion or fighting is seen in the client.

Taking Care of the Client with a Ventilator
• Be sure to carefully explain the purpose of the ventilator.
• Monitor breath sounds regularly (every 30 to 60 minutes).
• Measure arterial blood gases and pulse oximetry.
• Perform endotracheal suctioning when necessary.
• Ensure the client has a way to communicate (e.g. writing paper).
• Ensure the client can reach the call light.

Pulmonary Embolus

Key Points
• A clot, fat, or gaseous substance that obstructs the pulmonary artery.
• Clots can migrate from veins in the pelvis, legs, kidney or arms.
• Fat embolus: linked with long bone fractures.
• Air embolus: linked with the use of central lines.

- Amniotic embolus: either amniocentesis or abortion complication.
- Septic embolus: due to damaged heart valves, infected intravenous catheters, pelvic abscesses, and injections of illegal drugs.

Reduction of Pulmonary Embolus
- Antiembolism and pneumatic stockings.
- Ambulate postoperative patients.
- Avoid popliteal pressure.
- Monitor peripheral circulation.
- Regular changing of patients position.
- Check for heat, swelling, redness in IV sites.
- Refrain from leg muscle compression or massage.
- Ensure client does not cross their legs.
- Prevent client from smoking as much as possible.

Risk Factors
- Immobilization
- Fractures
- Trauma
- Clot formation history
- Smoking
- Pregnancy
- Estrogen therapy
- Oral contraceptives
- Lung cancer
- Advanced age
- Atrial fibrillation
- Artificial heart valves
- Sepsis
- Congestive heart failure.

Symptoms
- Pleuritic chest pain
- Fever

- Tachypnea
- Dyspnea
- Hypoxemia
- Syncope
- Hemoptysis
- Tachycardia
- Fluctutuations in T wave and S-T segments
- Hypotension
- Distended neck veins

Diagnosis: Involves chest x-rays which can show pulmonary infiltration, pulmonary angiography, and EGC (rules out myocardinal infarction).

Care and Treatment
- Putting client in high Fowler's sitting position.
- Providing oxygen using a mask.
- Providing chest pain medication.
- Thrombolytics.
- Antibiotics (clients with septic emboli).

Pneumothorax

Key Points
- Exposure of positive atmospheric pressure on the pleural space.
- Negative pressure is what normally keeps lungs inflated.
- Increase in intrathoracic pressure.
- Collapse in an area of the lung.

3 pneumothorax classifications:
Spontaneous pneumothorax - Not life threatening. Arises from a burst of a blister or bleb on the visceral pleura surface. Can also occur from chronic obstructive pulmonary disease.

Traumatic pneumothorax - Arises from chest trauma. Either the plural space is filled with air from the outside (open pneumothorax), or the pleural space is filled with air from the lung (closed pneumothorax). Both pose a serious threat to life.

Tension pneumothorax: - Arises from a leak of air in the chest wall or lung. Results in the collapse of the lung.

Assessment
• Reduced breath sounds
• Chest hyperresonance
• Tracheal deviation
• Tachypnea
• Cyanosis
• Pleuritic pain

Chest x-rays are used to confirm the condition.

Treatment
• Bore needle insertion (second intercostal space, mid-clavicular line on affected side).
• Chest tubes are inserted.
• Use of chest drainage system (water sealed).

Hemothorax

Key Points
• Build up of blood in the pleural space.
• Multiple causes, e.g. trauma, thoracic surgery.
• Blood creates pulmonary structure pressure.
• Collapse of alveoli.
• Decrease in gas exchange surface area.
• Cause hypoyvelemia.
• Severity depends on the amount of blood that is lost.

Assessment
- Reduced breath sounds.
- Respiratory distress.
- Pleural space blood accumulation.
- Percussion of the affected side creates dull sound.

Treatment

- Blood removal via chest tubes (anterior and posterior).
- Open thoracotomy for large blood loss.

Nurses should monitor the chest drainage system and intervene if complications occur.

Section 5: Emerging Respiratory Infections

There are certain diseases that have become more prevalent within the past two decades. Two examples of these are severe acute respiratory syndrome (SARS) and legionnaires' disease.

Severe Acute Respiratory Syndrome (SARS)

Key Points
- Pneumonia caused by a coronavirus, CoV.
- Coronavirus is responsible for around 1/3 of colds.
- SARS is spread by respiratory tract droplets.
- Possible transmission of the disease via contaminated water.
- 2 to 7 days incubation period.

Symptoms
- 100.4+ degrees fever
- Cough
- Headache
- Sore throat
- Shortness of breath
- Pneumonia seen in chest x-ray
- Possible development of acute respiratory distress.

Care of the Client
- Isolation.
- Quarantine.
- Negative pressure isolation room.
- Nurses should wear N95 masks and other contact precautions.

Legionnaires' Disease

Key Points
• Caused by the bacteria Legionella pneumophilia.
• The bacteria are found in water sources.
• Risk factors such as: immunosuppression, alcoholism, and pulmonary disease.
• Affects: lungs and other organs.

Symptoms
• Myalgia
• Headache
• Cough
• Fever
• Diarrhea
• Malaise
• Gastrointestinal issues

Care of the Client
• Same management to those that have pneumonia.
• Antibiotic therapy: Zithromax, Biaxin, Ilotycin, Levaquin.

Section 6: Important Concepts

In order to help you apply what you've learned into practice in your NCLEX test, this section will summarize the key concepts you should continuously revisit.

Key Terminology

- Acute respiratory failure
- Apnea
- Asthma
- Bronchitis
- Continuous positive airway pressure (CPAP)
- Cor pulmonale
- Cyanosis
- Dyspnea
- Emphysema
- Hemoptysis
- Hypoxemia
- Hypoxia
- Pleural effusion
- Pleurisy
- Pneumonia
- Pulmonary embolus
- Tachypnea

Key Diagnostic Tests for Respiratory Disorders

- CBC
- Chest x-ray
- Pulmonary function tests
- Lung scan
- Bronchoscopy

Section 7: Respiratory System Practice Questions & Rationales

1. A client has sustained injuries in a car accident. When the nurse is assessing the client, which injury has the greatest risk to the client?

a. Contusions of the lower legs
b. Fractures of the ribs
c. Lacerations of the face
d. Fractures of the humerus

Answer B is correct. A closed pneumothorax can be caused by fractures of the ribs. This is a life threatening situation which needs rapid detection and treatment. Answers A, C, and D are incorrect as they are not life threatening to the client.

2. Tension pneumothorax has which one of the following characteristics?

a. Tracheal deviation toward the unaffected side
b. Symmetry of the thorax and equal breath sounds
c. Tracheal deviation toward the affected side
d. Decreased heart rate and decreased respirations

Answer A is correct. When assessing a client, tension pneumothorax shows tracheal deviations towards the unaffected side. Answer B is incorrect because the thorax is asymmetrical and breath sounds are not present on the affected side. Answer C is incorrect because the deviation is toward the unaffected side, and not the affected side. Both the heart rate and respiratory rate are not decreased, which makes answer d incorrect.

3. A client with a closed chest drainage system is being cared for. What should the nurse do if the tubing gets disconnected from the system?

a. Instruct the client to perform the Valsalva maneuver
b. Elevate the tubing above the client's chest level
c. Form a water seal and obtain a new connector
d. Decrease the amount of suction being applied

Answer B is correct. A water seal should be formed by the nurse. They should remove the contaminated end, along with inserting another sterile connector. Answer A is incorrect because the Valsalva maneuver is utilized when the chest tube is being removed. The chest drainage system is kept below the chest level of the client, which makes answer B incorrect. The nurse cannot alter the amount of suction being applied without a doctor's order, therefore answer D is incorrect.

4. Theo-Dur (theophylline) is ordered by the physician for a client with emphysema. What is a side effects expected with this medication?

a. Palpitations
b. Mouth dryness
c. Hyperglycemia
d. Anemia

Answer A is correct. Palpitations, tremulousness, and restlessness are side effects that are expected from bronchodilators including theophylline. The other side effects are not associated with bronchodilators, therefore answers B, C, and D are incorrect.

5. For a client with pneumonia, which of the following conditions contraindicate the use of chest physiotherapy:

a. Rheumatoid arthritis
b. Diabetes mellitus
c. Recent abdominal cholecystectomy
d. Emphysema

Answer B is correct. Contraindications for chest physiotherapy are recent abdominal or thoracic surgery. Diabetes mellitus, rheumatoid arthritis, or emphysema, are not contraindicated for the use of chest physiotherapy, thus answers A, C, and D are incorrect.

6. A client's tuberculosis skin test is being interpreted by the nurse. A false positive tuberculosis skin test is caused by which one of the following factors:

a. Vaccination with a live virus
b. Weakened immune system
c. Poor testing technique
d. BCG vaccine inoculation

Answer D is correct. A BCG vaccine inoculation will cause a false positive tuberculosis skin test. Answers A, B, and C are factors that can cause a false negative tuberculosis skin test, therefore these answers are incorrect.

7. A client has pulmonary fibrosis, and Cytoxan (cyclophosphamide) has been ordered by the physician.

Which one of the following instructions should be given to the client by the nurse?

a. Notify the doctor of a sore throat or fever
b. Walk 20 minutes a day to maintain muscle strength
c. Expect a reddish discoloration of her urine
d. Eat smaller, more frequent meals

Answer A is correct. Any symptoms linked with infection should be reported. This is because Cytoxan is an immunosuppressive drug. Answers b and D are incorrect because the are not associated with the use of Cytoxan. Hemorrhagic cystitis can be experience by a client taking Cytoxan as result of too little fluid intake, however this is not expected, so answer C is incorrect.

8. There is a limited supply of the influenza vaccine available for use by the physician. Who should be given priority for receiving the influenza immunization?

a. An elementary school teacher
b. An office worker
c. A resident in a nursing home
d. A local firefighter

Answer C is correct. When supplies are limited, priority for the influenza vaccine should be given to those aged 65+ and clients with chronic conditions. Answers A, B, and D are incorrect: they are not given priority in receiving the vaccine.

9. A client has tuberculosis, and Pyrazinamide is ordered by the physician. What should the nurse instruct the client to do?

a. Schedule frequent eye exams
b. Increase his fluid intake
c. Expect red discoloration of his urine
d. Expect dizziness and ringing in his ears

Answer b is correct. The client should increase their fluid intake because gout-like symptoms can be caused by the use of pyrazinamide. Answers A, C, and D are incorrect: they are linked with other antitubercular medications.

10. A client with Legionnaires' disease is being cared for by the nurse. When caring for the client, which one of the following isolation types should the nurse use?

a. Droplet precautions
b. No isolation precautions are needed
c. Airborne precautions
d. Contact precautions

Answer B is correct. There is no evidence of human to human transmission, therefore no isolation precautions are necessary. The other precautions are not required in the care of those with Legionnaires' disease, therefore answers A, C, and D are incorrect.

11. The nurse discovers that a client has a barrel chest when conducting an assessment on a client with emphysema. The client's chest alterations is a result of which of the following:

a. Distal alveoli collapse
b. Long term chronic hypoxia
c. Hyperinflation of the lungs
d. Accessory muscle use

Answer C is correct. A barrel chest develops for clients with emphysema as a result air being trapped in the lungs - this causes them to hyperinflate. Although answers B and D are incorrect even though they are common for clients with emphysema. Answer A is incorrect because this does not occur in emphysema.

12. The nurse realizes that a client with chronic obstructive pulmonary disease (COPD) shows more dyspnea in a particular positioning. Which of the following positions is best to relieve the client's dyspnea?

a. Standing or sitting upright
b. Lying supine with a single pillow
c. Side lying with the head elevated
d. Lying with head slightly lowered

Answer A is correct. Breathing is more difficult when a client is laying down with chronic obstructive pulmonary disease. Standing or sitting upright makes their respiratory process better. Their bed can also be positioned in high Fowler's position. Answers B, C, and D are incorrect as the do not relieve the client's dyspnea.

13. A nurse is evaluating the chart of a client with long standing lung disease. They should pay particular attention to which of the following pulmonary function test results:

a. Residual volume
b. Total lung capacity
c. Functional residual capacity
d. FEV1/FVC ratio

Answer D is correct. Disease progression is indicated by the FEV1/FVC ratio. The ratio of FEV1 to FVC becomes smaller as COPD gets worse. Answers A and B are incorrect because they indicate loss of elastic recoil as a result of narrowing and obstruction of the airway. Functional residual capacity is increased in clients with obstructive bronchitis, therefore answer C is incorrect.

14. O2 at 3 liters per minute via nasal cannula is ordered by the physician. When a client has COPD, O2 amounts larger than 3 liters per minute are contraindicated for which of the following reasons:

a. Hypoxic drive is needed for breathing.
b. Higher concentrations result in severe headache.
c. Hypercapnic drive is necessary for breathing.
 d. Higher levels will be required later to raise the pO2.

Answer A is correct. In clients with COPD, the stimulation of respiratory effort occurs due to hypoxemia. Answers C and D are incorrect because higher levels would prevent the client from the power to breathe. Answer B is a statement that is incorrect.

15. A client is taking a bronchodilator. They inform the nurse that when they are discharged they are going to begin a smoking cessation. If their smoking pattern changes, they should inform the doctor because they will:

a. Require an increase in antitussive medication
b. Need his medication dosage adjusted
c. No longer need annual influenza immunization
d. Not derive as much benefit from inhaler use

Answer B is correct.
The amount of meditation needed will be impacted when smoking patterns are changed, and these should be discussed with the physician. Clients with COPD are placed not placed on antitussives, but on expectorants, therefor answer A is incorrect. Annual influenza vaccinations are recommended for all clients with lung disease, therefore answer C is incorrect. Answer D is incorrect because inhaler benefits are expected to increase when the client stops smoking.

16. A client's serum aminophylline level is 17mcg/mL as indicated by lab results. The nurse notes that the aminophylline level is:

a. Too high and should be reported
b. Questionable and should be repeated
c. Within therapeutic range
d. Too low to be therapeutic

Answer C is correct. Aminophylline between 10–20 mcg/ml is within therapeutic range. Answers A and D are incorrect. There is nothing to suggest that the results are questionable, therefor answer B is incorrect.

17. A client with emphysema has experienced a gain in morning weight of 5 pounds in less than 7 days. Their oral intake has been modest. What complication of COPD may be responsible for the client's weight gain?

a. Polycythemia
b. Compensated acidosis
c. Left ventricular failure

d. Cor pulmonale

Answer D is correct. A possible complication of emphysema is Cor pulmonale (right sided heart failure) . Answers A and B are not responsible for weight gain. Answer C would be indicated in pulmonary edema, therefore it is incorrect.

18. The nurse is teaching a client the proper way of using a metered dose inhaler. Which of the following actions suggests the client requires additional guidance?

a. The client takes a deep breath while depressing the inhaler.
b. The client waits 15 seconds before using the inhaler a second time.
c. The client places the inhaler two fingers from the mouth.
d. The client exhales slowly using purse lipped breathing.

Answer B is correct. The inhaler should only be used a second time after the client has waited 60 seconds, therefore this needs to be correctly taught to the client. Answers A, C, and D indicate that the client understands the correct use of the inhaler.

19. Weight loss for a client with COPD may occur, even with a significant intake of calories. When discussing with the client the ways they can maintain weight, what should the nurse advise the client to do?

a. Continue the same caloric intake and increase the amount of fat intake
b. Increase his activity level to stimulate his appetite
c. Decrease the amount of complex carbohydrates while increasing calories, protein, vitamins, and minerals

d. Increase the amount of complex carbohydrates and decrease the amount of fat intake

Answer C is correct. A greater volume of calories, protein, minerals and vitamins are needed for a client with COPD. The client requires more calories but not more fat, therefore answer A is incorrect. Answer B is incorrect - this will create greater weight loss. Answer D will create excess acid production, along with a greater respiratory workload.

20. The client has been given garamycin 65 mg IVPB regularly every 8 hours for the past 6 days. An adverse reaction to the medication is indicated by which lab result?

a. WBC 7500
b. Serum creatinine 2.0
c. Serum glucose 92
d. Protein 3.5

Answer B is correct. Renal impairment is indicated by the elevated serum creatinine. The other answers are within standard limits.

21. Chest physiotherapy has been ordered for a client with chronic obstructive lung disease. What should the nurse give priority to when performing chest physiotherapy?

a. Covering the client's chest with a towel
b. Placing the client in a prone position
c. Making sure that the client's face is visible
d. Beginning percussion in the lower lobes

Answer C is correct. A mucus plug could obstruct the airway that could prevent the client from speaking, therefore the nurse should be able to see the client's face when performing percussion. Answers A, B, and D are incorrect because they do not take priority over keeping the airway open.

22. A client with acute respiratory distress syndrome (ARDS) is admitted to the intensive care unit. Which of the following statements applies to acute respiratory distress syndrome?

a. A direct cause of the disorder is left-sided heart failure
b. Only clients with chronic pulmonary disease are affected by the disorder
c. The disorder is characterized by refractory hypoxemia
d. The disorder responds very favorably to surfactant replacement

Answer C is correct. ARDS is distinguished by the appearance of 'ground glass' infiltrates. These reduce gas exchange in the lungs lead to refractory hypoxemia. Answers A, B, and D are statements that are incorrect.

23. A client has a three-chamber chest drainage system. While evaluating the client, the nurse notes that there is no fluctuation of the level of fluid in the second chamber. Which of the following actions is suitable for the nurse to take:

a. Empty the fluid from the second chamber
b. Determine if the suction is working correctly
c. Call the doctor and prepare to change systems
d. Increase the amount of suction applied

Answer B is correct. It is possible that the suction not working correctly is causing the absence of fluctuation in the second chamber. The nurse should work out whether this is the cause. Obstruction in the tubing or reinflation of the lung are other possible causes of missing fluctuation in the water seal chamber. There should be no removal of fluid from the chamber, therefore answer A is incorrect. Answer C is incorrect - there are no signs that indicate the doctor needs to be informed or that there needs to be another insertion of the chest tube. Without a doctors consent, the nurse cannot increase the amount of suction, therefore answer D is incorrect.

24. Purse-lipped breathing is being taught to a 10 year old client with cystic fibrosis. Which of the following would be an effective activity for helping the child learn the technique?

a. Using an incentive spirometer three times a day
b. Doing sit-ups to strengthen abdominal muscles
c. Blowing a ping pong ball across a table
d. Blowing out a lit candle

Answer C is correct. Purse lipped breathing can be effectively taught by getting the client do engage in activities such as blowing a ping pong ball across the table - this can be turned into a game for a child. Answer A is incorrect because this does not focus on purse lipped breathing but deeper breathing. Answer C would fail to teach purse lipped breathing. Answer D is incorrect because blowing out a candle is too deep a breath for purse lipped breathing.

25. A client has PCP pneumonia. An infusion of Pentam (pentamidine) is being prepared to be administered by the

nurse. An adverse reaction to the medication is indicated by which lab finding?

a. WBC 7500/cu. mm
b. Platelets 200,000/cu. mm
c. Neutrophils 52%
d. RBC 2,500,000/cu. mm

Answer D is correct. Anemia is indicated by the client's RBC. Anemia, thrombocytopenia, and nephrotoxicity are adverse reactions to pentamidine. Answers A, B, and C are incorrect because they are within the normal range.

26. A client with emphysema is being given dietary teaching. The teaching has been effective, which statement made by the client indicates this?

a. "Smaller, more frequent meals with increased protein and fat will be best."
b. "I will need to restrict the amount of fluids I drink each day."
c. "I should supplement my meals with high-protein milkshakes."
d. "Consuming hot meals will be best since I will feel less full after eating."

Answer A is correct. Eating 5-6 meals a day will best meet the needs of a client with emphysema. On top of this, these meals should contain increased calories, fat, and protein. The client needs to take in a greater amount of fluid to liquefy secretions, therefore answer B is incorrect. Answer C is incorrect because the client needs to stay away from drinks that will thicken secretions, such as milk. Consuming hot foods gives a greater sense of fullness, therefore answer D is incorrect.

27. The risk of developing a pulmonary embolus is greatest for which one of the following:

a. 21-year-old male who has a fractured radius
b. 55-year-old male with type II diabetes mellitus
c. 40-year-old female who had a total hysterectomy

d. 65-year-old female with hyperthyroidism

Answer C is correct. Surgery within the last three months, immobilization, stroke, DVT history, and malignancy are common factors that pose a risk for the development of pulmonary embolus. Answers A, B, and D are incorrect because they are not linked with an greater risk of pulmonary embolus.

28. The nurse should give priority to which of the following when providing care for a client with a new tracheostomy:

a. Using aseptic technique when cleaning the tracheostomy
b. Oxygenating the client with 100% oxygen before suctioning
c. Ensuring a snug fit between the tracheostomy ties and the neck
d. Changing the disposable inner cannula every 48 hours

Answer B is correct. To prevent hypoxia, the client should be given 100% oxygen before suctioning. A sterile (not aseptic) technique is utilized when giving care for a new tracheostomy, therefore answer A is incorrect. Answer C is incorrect - two fingers should be able to be placed between the tracheostomy ties and the client's neck. Answer D is incorrect because a new tracheostomy inner cannula should be changed regularly every 12–24 hours.

29. A prescription for prednisone is given to a client being discharged with sarcoidosis. The discharge teaching that the client receives should include which one of the following instructions:

a. Limit the intake of foods high in potassium.
b. Increase the intake of foods high in sodium.
c. Take the medication at bedtime.
d. Notify the physician if you have a fever or sore throat.

Answer D is correct. There is an increased risk of infection for clients taking glucocortiocoids such as prednisone. The early signs of infection are fever and sore throat are - these need to be reported to the physician. Answer A is incorrect because the client requires an intake of foods that are rich in potassium. The client needs to decrease the intake of foods high in sodium to decrease fluid retention, therefore answer B is incorrect. Medication needs to be taken every day before 9AM, therefore answer C is incorrect.

30. A client sustained blunt chest trauma to the right rib cage. While assessing the client, the nurse observes reduced breath sounds on the affected side with tracheal deviation toward the unaffected side. What should the nurse prepare to assist with?

a. Endotracheal intubation
b. Chest tube insertion
c. Chest physiotherapy
d. Venopuncture for ABGs

Answer B is correct. Signs of a pneumothorax are being shown by the client. The nurse should prepare to provide assistance for chest tube insertion. There are no signs of the need for endotracheal intubation, therefore answer A is incorrect. Answer C is incorrect because chest physiotherapy is contraindicated for those with thoracic trauma. Answer D is incorrect because ABGs are not obtained on venous blood, but arterial blood.

31. The risk of Legionnaire's disease is greatest for which one of the following clients:

a. 60-year-old coal miner who has a 2 PPD smoking history
b. 21-year-old college freshman who lives in a dormitory
c. 35-year-old automobile salesman who works outside
d. 55-year-old teacher who frequently travels abroad

Answer A is correct. Those most susceptible to Legionnaire's disease are smokers, older adults, and clients with chronic disease. Other factors are a client's age, occupation, and whether they smoke. Answers B, C, and D are incorrect because these clients are not at increased risk for Legionnaire's disease.

32. A client is admitted with pulmonary tuberculosis. Which of the following transmission-based precautions should the nurse take for this client?

a. Droplet precautions
b. Contact precautions
c. Airborne precautions
d. Standard precautions

Answer C is correct. Droplets from the respiratory tract spread the organism that causes tuberculosis. Droplets are suspended in the air for a number of hours - airborne precautions are important for pulmonary tuberculosis care. Nurses should wear a respirator mask (N-95 or HEPA mask) before entering the room that the client is in. Answers A, B, and D are incorrect because they are not utilized to stop the spread of tuberculosis.

33. Preparation for the ambulation of a client with a closed chest drainage system is taking place. What should the nurse do to promote drainage and also prevent reflux?

a. Keep the drainage system lower than the chest
b. Clamp the tubing while the client is out of bed
c. Empty the drainage system before ambulating
d. Keep the drainage system level with the insertion site

Answer A is correct. The chest drainage system should be kept below the level of the chest, in order to promote drainage and prevent reflux. Answers B, C, and D are incorrect - closed-chest drainage systems should not be managed in any of these ways.

34. When instructing a client to use a dry-powder inhaler, which one of the following statements made by the client suggests a need for further teaching?

a. "I will keep the inhaler level with the mouthpiece end facing down."
b. "I will inhale deeply through my mouth for 2–3 seconds."
c. "I will brush my teeth after I finish using the inhaler."
d. "I will keep the inhaler stored in the refrigerator."

Answer D is correct. A clean, dry location is where the dry-powder inhaler should be stored. It should not be stored in a refrigerator, therefore the nurse should give the client further instruction and advise them on the best place to store the inhaler. Answers A, B, and C are incorrect because they show a proper understanding of the correct use of the dry powder inhaler.

35. Myambutol (ethambutol) is ordered by the physician as part of a four-drug regimen for treating a tuberculosis client. Which of the following side effects are associated with ethambutol use?

a. Red discoloration of the urine
b. Changes in color perception
c. Deficiency of pyridoxine (B6)
d. Swollen, painful joints

Answer B is correct. A change in vision and color perception is a side effect of ethambutol. The client should have a visual exam before the start of therapy to establish a baseline, along with regular eye examinations planned throughout the treatment. Red Urine discoloration is a side effect of rifampin, therefore answer A is incorrect. Deficiency of pyridoxine (B6) is a side effect associated with isoniazid, therefore answer C is incorrect. Answer D is incorrect as swollen and painful joints are a pyrazinamide side effect.

36. A client has emphysema. A red blood cell count of 8,000,000/cu mm in their CBC. What does the nurse recognize the client has an increased risk for based on the client's lab results?

a. Hemorrhagic stroke

b. Hospital-acquired pneumonia
c. Thrombus formation
d. Prolonged bleeding

Answer C is correct. An elevation in red blood cells in the client's CBC - this increases the client's thrombus formation risk. Answers A and D are incorrect because they are not linked with an rise in the number of red blood cells, but with a fall in the number of platelets. Answer B is incorrect because hospital-acquired pneumonia is not related to the increased number of red blood cells.

37. Cytoxan (cyclophosphamide) is prescribed for a client with pulmonary fibrosis. Which of the following should the nurse instruct the client to do:

a. Take the medication with grapefruit juice to make it more digestible
b. Drink 10 to 12 glasses of water a day while taking the medication
c. Refrain from the use of acetaminophen while taking the medication
d. Take the medication with meals or a snack

Answer B is correct. To reduce the risk of developing hemorrhagic cystitis, the nurse should advise the client to drink 10 to 12 glasses of water a day. Answer A is incorrect because this will not make the medication more digestible. The client can continue to use acetaminophen, therefore answer C is incorrect. Answer D is incorrect because the medication should be not been taken with food, but taken on an empty stomach.

38. The nurse is preparing to administer a PPD skin test. The nurse discovers that the client was given the BCG vaccine whilst living in a foreign country. Which of the following actions should the nurse take:

a. Administer the PPD skin test
b. Obtain a sputum specimen
c. Request an order for isoniazid
d. Obtain an order for a chest x-ray

Answer D is correct. Prior vaccination with the BCG vaccine will lead the client to show a false positive result on the PPD skin test, so the nurse should make an order for a chest x-ray. Giving the PPD skin test to this client would result in a false positive result, therefore answer A is incorrect. Answer B is incorrect because the client requires a chest x-ray and only sputum if necessary. Answer C is false because the client should be evaluated with a chest x-ray first.

39. A client has pleural effusion, and has developed subcutaneous emphysema after thoracentesis. Which of the following findings is a characteristic of subcutaneous emphysema?

a. Auscultation of reduced breath sounds on the affected side
b. Crackling sensation noted in the skin near the puncture site
c. Paradoxical movement of the chest with inhalation and exhalation
d. Chest asymmetry and distended neck veins on the opposite side

Answer B is correct. Subcutaneous emphysema results as a result of air entering the subcutaneous tissue. This creates a crackling sensation when the area is examined. Answer A is incorrect - this is a description of a pneumothorax. Answer C is incorrect - this is a description of a flail chest. Answer D is incorrect - this is a description of a tension pneumothorax.

40. A nurse is arranging care for a client on a ventilator. Which of the following interventions gives the client the greatest sense of control over their environment?

a. Allowing visits with his family and friends
b. Explaining procedures before they are done
c. Keeping the call light within reach
d. Providing pencil and writing paper

Answer C is correct. The best way of allowing the client control over their environment is keeping the call light within reach. Answer A is incorrect because it decreases their isolation but does not provide them with more control over their environment. Answer B is incorrect because this is a situation in which the nurse is in control. Answer D gives a way for the client to communicate but no extra control, therefore this answer is incorrect.

41. A client has community-acquired pneumonia. They have been receiving intravenous Geopen (carbenicillin). Which of the following findings should alert the nurse to drug reaction that is adverse?

a. Diarrhea containing blood and mucus
b. Burning at the infusion site
c. Loss of appetite
d. Headache and myalgia

Answer A is correct. Diarrhea stools that contain blood indicate pseudomembraneous colitis - this is an adverse reaction to antibiotic therapy. Answer B is incorrect because burning at the infusion site is not linked with an adverse drug reaction. Answers C and D are incorrect - they are not symptoms associated with the prescribed drug, but symptoms associated with the illness.

42. The suction setting should be set between which of the following when performing endotracheal suctioning:

a. 20 mm Hg and 50 mm Hg
b. 70 mm Hg and 100 mm Hg
c. 130 mm Hg and 170 mm Hg
d. 80 mm Hg and 120 mm Hg

Answer D is correct. The suction should be set between 80 mm Hg and 120 mm Hg. The suction settings for Answers A and B are too low. Answer C is incorrect - this is a suction setting that is too high.

43. When administering an annual influenza vaccine, which of the following allergies should the nurse question the client about?

a. Milk
b. Eggs
c. Shellfish
d. Nuts

Answer A is correct. Eggs because eggs are used in the manufacturing of the influenza vaccination, therefore the client should be questioned for egg allergies. Answers A, C, and D are incorrect because they not associated with the manufacturing of the influenza vaccine.

44. An elderly client has chronic obstructive lung disease, and pulse oximetry has been ordered. Where is the best probe placement location for the client:

a. Toe
b. Earlobe
c. Finger
d. Chest

Answer B is correct. The earlobe is is least affected by decreased blood flow, so this is the best location for probe placement. Answers A and B are incorrect because decreased flow of blood to the fingers and toes obstructs with pulse oximetry readings. the chest is not a suitable site for placement, therefore answer D is incorrect.

45. A client with primary pulmonary hypertension who has developed cor pulmonale is being cared for by the nurse. Which of the following findings is a characteristic of a client with cor pulmonale?

a. Expectoration of frothy, pink sputum
b. Decreased daytime voiding
c. Hacking nighttime cough
d. Edema of the legs and sacrum

Answer D is correct. Edema of the legs and sacrum is a frequent finding associated with cor pulmonale (right sided heart failure). Answers A, B, and C are incorrect because they are associated symptoms of left sided heart failure.

46. A client's pulmonary artery pressure is being evaluated by the nurse. The nurse is knows that this test measures:

a. The systolic, diastolic, and mean pressure of the pulmonary artery
b. Pressure in the left ventricle
c. The pressure in the pulmonary veins
d. The pressure in the right ventricle

Answer A is correct. The pressure throughout the diastole, systole, and mean pressure in the pulmonary artery will be measured by the pulmonary artery pressure. Answers B, C, and D are incorrect as it will not measure the pressure in the left ventricle, right ventricle pressure, or the pulmonary vein pressure.

47. A client with chronic obstructive pulmonary disease is admitted. It is revealed in blood gases that pH 7.36, CO2 45, O2 84, bicarb 28. What would the nurse would assess the client to be in?

a. Uncompensated acidosis
b. Compensated respiratory acidosis
c. Compensated alkalosis
d. Uncompensated metabolic acidosis

Answer B is correct. Compensated metabolic acidosis is being experienced by the client. The pH is on the acidic side, it is within the standard range, however it is lower than 7.40. The CO2 level is raised, the oxygen level is below standard, and the bicarb level is slightly increased. The pH will be the inverse of the CO2 and bicarb levels in respiratory disorders. This means that the CO2 and bicarb levels will be elevated if the level of pH is low. Answers A, C, and D are incorrect - they do not fall into the scope of symptoms.

48. A client with lung cancer is having a removal of the left lower lobe of the lung. Which of the following post-operative measures would generally be included in the schedule?

a. A tracheostomy
b. A Swan Ganz Monitor
c. Percussion vibration and drainage
d. Closed chest drainage

Answer D is correct. The client with a lung resection will have chest tubes, along with a device for drainage-collection. They will likely not have a tracheostomy or Swanz Ganz monitoring, and not have an plan for vibration, percussion, or drainage. Therefore, answers A, B, and C are incorrect.

49. An eight-year-old child admitted with asthma is being cared for by the nurse. Durin the morning rounds, the nurse finds an O2 sat of 78%. Which action should the nurse take first?

a. Notify the physician
b. Apply oxygen
c. Do nothing; this is a normal O2 sat for a nine-year-old
d. Assess the child's pulse

Answer C is correct. Remember Airway, Breathing, Circulation (ABC's) when you answering this question. Oxygen should be applied to increase the child's oxygen saturation, before notifying the physician or monitoring the child's pulse. 92% to 100% is the normal oxygen saturation for a child. Although answer A is important, it is not the priority. Answer B is not an appropriate action, and answer D should not be the primary action taken.

50. A 9-year-old is receiving treatment for asthma . Which of the following should the nurse check before administering Theodur:
a. Urinary output
b. Blood pressure
c. Temperature
d. Pulse

Answer D is correct. As Theodur is a bronchodilator, a side effect of it is tachycardia - this makes checking the pulse is important. Extreme tachycardia needs to be reported to the doctor. Answers A, B, and D are unnecessary.

51. A client admitted with acute laryngotracheobronchitis (LTB) is being cared for by the nurse. Which of the following should the nurse have available, due to the possibility of complete obstruction of the airway?

a. Emergency intubation equipment
b. Intravenous access supplies
c. Intravenous fluid-administration pump
d. Supplemental oxygen

Answer A is correct. Emergency intubation equipment should always be kept at the bedside. This is for a child with LTB and the associated possibility of complete obstruction of the airway. Answers B, C, and D are incorrect because intravenous supplies and fluid will not treat an obstruction, neither will supplemental oxygen.

52. Respirations by a post-operative client have fallen from 14 to 6 breaths per minute. Per standing order, the nurse administers Narcan (naloxone). What should the nurse assess the client for following administration of the medication?

a. Pupillary changes
b. Projectile vomiting
c. Sudden, intense pain
d. Wheezing respirations

Answer C is correct. The client will experience intense and sudden pain because Narcan (narcotic antagonist) blocks the effects of the client's pain medication. Answers A, B, and D are incorrect because they are not related to the condition of the client or Narcan administration.

53. Which of the following obstetrical clients is the most likely to have an child with respiratory distress syndrome?

a. A 24-year-old with a history of diabetes mellitus
b. A 28-year-old with a history of alcohol use during the pregnancy
c. A 30-year-old with a history of smoking during the pregnancy
d. A 32-year-old with a history of pregnancy-induced hypertension

Answer A is correct. Those with a history of diabetes are the most likely to deliver a preterm large for gestational age baby. These newborns are often unable to prevent respiratory distress syndrome because they often lack sufficient surfactant levels. Answers B, C, and D are incorrect because they are not as likely to have newborns with respiratory distress syndrome.

54. Which of the following is a primary physiological alteration in asthma development:

a. Bronchiolar inflammation and dyspnea
b. Hypersecretion of abnormally viscous mucus
c. Spasm of bronchiolar smooth muscle
d. Infectious processes causing mucosal edema

Answer C is correct. Asthma is the occurrence of bronchiolar spasms. Either allergies or anxiety can stimulate these spasms. Answer A is incorrect because inflammation is not the primary physiological alteration. Answer B is incorrect because the production of abnormally viscous mucus is not a primary alteration. Infection is not primary to asthma which makes Answer C incorrect.

55. Which of the following assessment findings indicate a chronic respiratory problem in a client with COPD?

a. Wheezing on exhalation
b. Clubbing of fingers
c. Productive cough
d. Generalized cyanosis

Answer B is correct. The clinical indication of clubbing of the fingers occurs over a period of time. This indicates that the condition not acute, but chronic. Answers A, C, and D are incorrect because they are not associated with chronicity.

56. A client with chronic airway disease is being cared for by the nurse. Which of the following changes are reversible in the following associated disorders?

a. Bronchiectasis
b. Emphysema
c. Asthma
d. Chronic bronchitis

Answer C is correct. The only disorder that is reversible spontaneously or with treatment is Asthma. Answers A, B, and D are incorrect because they can generate irreversible damage to parts of the respiratory system.

57. Shortness of breath, pain upon deep breathing, and hemoptysis are being experienced by a a client with a fractured leg. Which of the following do these clinical manifestations indicate to the nurse:

a. Pulmonary embolus
b. Congestive heart failure
c. Adult respiratory distress syndrome
d. Tension pneumothorax

Answer A is correct. A key symptom of a pulmonary embolus is Hemoptysis, the client's leg fracture history and other clinical manifestations produce this conclusion. Answers B, C, and D are incorrect because the client's clinical manifestations are not associated with them.

58. A client with multiple rib fractures and a pulmonary contusion is being cared for by the nurse in the emergency room. A respiratory rate of 38 is revealed in assessment, along with a heart rate of 136, and restlessness. Which of

the following associated assessment findings would require intervention immediately?

a. Occasional small amounts of hemoptysis
b. Subcutaneous air and absent breath sounds
c. Midline trachea with wheezing on auscultation
d. Pain when breathing deeply, with rales in the upper lobes

Answer B is correct. A pneumothorax is indicated by the absence of breath sounds and subcutaneous air, increased heart rate, dyspnea, and restlessness - therefore immediate intervention is necessary. Answer A is incorrect because this would be expected with pulmonary contusion. Answer D is incorrect because this would be associated with fractured ribs. Answer C is incorrect - the midline trachea is an expected finding.

59. A client is being assessed for tactile fremitus by the nurse. Which diagnoses would be most expected to show a decrease in tactile fremitus?

a. Bronchial pneumonia
b. Tuberculosis
c. Lung tumor
d. Emphysema

Answer D is correct. Tactile fremitus is observed by having the client to repeat terms such as number while the nurse's hands move down the thorax. Air does not conduct sound as well as a solid substance, therefore fremitus is increased with a solid substance. As with emphysema, fremitus is decreased when air is present. Answers A and C are incorrect because these are solid-tissue illnesses that would produce an increase in tactile fremitus. Bronchopneumonia generally develops with tuberculosis which causes increased fremitus, therefore answer answer A is incorrect.

60. A client with emphysema has recently been admitted by the nurse. Hypoxia is indicated by arterial blood gas. Which of the following physician prescriptions would be implemented by the nurse for the best improvement in hypoxia in the client?

a. Start oxygen at 2L/min.
b. Elevate the head of the bed 45°.
c. Encourage diaphragmatic breathing.
d. Initiate an Alupent nebulizer treatment.

Answer A is correct. The best means to correct hypoxia is the delivery of oxygen. Answers C, and D are incorrect because although they would also likely improve hypoxia, oxygen is the prescription that would provide instant relief.

61. There is an order for intravenous ampicillin for a client that has been admitted for treatment of bacterial pneumonia. Which of the following specimens should be obtained before administering the medication:

a. Routine urinalysis
b. Complete blood count
c. Sputum for culture and sensitivity
d. Serum electrolytes

Answer C is correct. In order to determine whether the organism is sensitive to the medication prescribed, sputum specimen for culture and sensitivity should be taken before the antibiotic is administered. Answers A, B, and D are incorrect because routine urinalysis, complete blood count, and serum electrolytes can be taken after the medication is administered.

62. A group of senior citizens are being taught healthful lifestyles by a community health nurse. The nurse should be aware that the biggest cause of death in persons 65+ is:

a. Chronic pulmonary disease
b. Diabetes mellitus
c. Heart disease
d. Pneumonia

Answer C is correct. Heart disease is the largest cause of death in persons 65 and older, according to the National Center for Health Statistics. Answer A is incorrect because chronic pulmonary disease is the ranked the forth cause of death for those in this age group. Answers B and D are incorrect because diabetes mellitus is ranked sixth and pneumonia is ranked fifth.

63. Which of the following types of endotracheal tube is recommended by the Centers for Disease Control (CDC) for decreasing the risk of ventilator-associated pneumonia?

a. CASS
b. Uncuffed
c. Fenestrated
d. Nasotracheal

Answer A is correct. The continuous aspiration of subglottic secretions (CASS) tube includes an evacuation port above the cuff, which makes it possible to remove secretions above the cuff. Answer B is incorrect because the use of an uncuffed tube increases the incidence of ventilator pneumonia by allowing aspiration of secretions. Answer C is incorrect because the fenestrated tube has openings that elevate the risk of pneumonia. Nasotracheal does not refer to a type of tube, but one of the routes for inserting an endotracheal tube, therefore answer D is incorrect.

64. A child is a family contact to the client that has tuberculosis. A prescription of Isoniazid (INH) has been provided for the client. Which of the following is the correct amount of time that the medication should be taken:

a. Six months
b. Three months
c. One year
d. Two years

Answer A is correct. Those living in the same household should take INH for approximately six months. Any time shorter or longer than this is not the correct amount of time to take the medication, therefore answers B, C, and D are incorrect.

65. An order for a sweat test is do be done on a child with a history of respiratory infections. Which of the following findings would be positive for cystic fibrosis?

a. A serum sodium of 135meq/L
b. A potassium of 4.5meq/L
c. A sweat analysis of 69 meq/L
d. A calcium of 8mg/dL

Answer C is correct. Cystic fibrosis is a exocrine glands disease. A child with cystic fibrosis will be salty, therefore a sweat test result of 60meq/L and higher is considered positive. Answers A, B, and D are incorrect because these test results would be within the standard range.

66. A client with a pulmonary embolis has Heparin ordered for them. Which of the following statements would indicate an inadequate understanding of the medication?

a. "I will need to aspirate when I give Heparin."
b. "I will administer the medication 1-2 inches away from the umbilicus."
c. "I will administer the medication in the abdomen."
d. "I will check the PTT before administering the medication."

Answer D is correct. This shows a lack of understanding of the correct method of administering heparin. A, B, and C are incorrect because they indicate a correct understanding.

67. Rifampin 600mg po is being taken daily by the client to treat their tuberculosis. Which of the following actions indicates a proper understanding of the medication:

a. Telling the client that the medication will need to be taken with juice
b. Telling the client to take the medication before going to bed at night
c. Telling the client that the medication will change the color of the urine
d. Telling the client to take the medication if night sweats occur

Answer C is correct. The color of urine and body fluid can be changed by rifampin. The client will likely be concerned about this, so it is best to teach the client about these changes. Answer A is incorrect because it is not unnecessary. Answer B is incorrect. Answer D is false - during the course of treatment, this medication should be taken regularly.

68. Emphysema and cor pulmonale have been diagnosed for a client. Which of the following findings are characteristics of cor pulmonale:

a. Hypoxia, shortness of breath, and exertional fatigue
b. Edema of the lower extremities and distended neck veins
c. Weight loss, increased RBC, and fever
d. Rales, edema, and enlarged spleen

Answer B is correct. Cor pulmonale (right-sided heart failure) is distinguished by edema of the legs and feet, distended neck veins, and an enlarged liver. Answer A is incorrect because these are symptoms associated with left-sided heart failure and pulmonary edema. Answer C is incorrect because it is not relevant to the question. Answer D does not relate to cor pulmonale, therfore it is incorrect.

69. A client begins to fight the ventilator on a mechanical ventilator. Which of the following medications will be ordered for the client:

a. Pavulon (pancuronium bromide)
b. Sublimaze (fentanyl)
c. Versed (midazolam)
d. Atarax (hydroxyzine)

Answer A is correct. Pavulon is a neuromuscular blocking agent that paralyzes skeletal muscles - this makes it impossible for the client to fight the ventilator. Answer B is incorrect because sublimaze is an analgesic used to control operative pain. Answer C is incorrect because versed is a benzodiazepine used to produce conscious sedation. Atarax is used to treat post-operative nausea, therefore answer D is incorrect.

70. Inhalation therapy with Pulmozyme (dornase alfa) is being used as a treatment for a child with cystic fibrosis. What is a side effect of this mediation?

a. Sore throat
b. Weight gain
c. Hair loss
d. Brittle nails

Answer A is correct. Sore throat, laryngitis and hoarseness are side effects of Pulmozyme. Answers B, C, and D are incorrect because they not associated with Pulmozyme.

71. Intravenous aminophylline is being given to a client with emphysema. Which level of aminophylline is associated with signs of toxicity?

a. 5 micrograms/mL
b. 10 micrograms/mL
c. 20 micrograms/mL
d. 25 micrograms/mL

Answer D is correct. 10–20 micrograms/mL is the therapeutic range for aminophylline. Levels that are higher than 20 micrograms/mL can generate signs of toxicity. Answer A is false because it is too low to be therapeutic. Answers B and C are incorrect because they are within the therapeutic range.

72. Which of the following findings best indicates that a client with ineffective airway clearance needs suctioning?

a. Oxygen saturation
b. Breath sounds
c. Respiratory rate
d. Arterial blood gases

Answer B is correct. The need for suctioning in the client with ineffective airway clearance is best indicated in changes in breath sounds. Answers A, C, and D are incorrect - they can be changed by other conditions.

73. Symptoms of respiratory distress are developed by a client with an esophageal tamponade, including inspiratory stridor. What should the nurse give priority to?

a. Removing the tube after deflating the balloons
b. Applying oxygen at 4L via nasal cannula
c. Elevating the head of the bed to 45°
d. Increasing the pressure in the esophageal balloon

Answer A is correct. The most likely cause of respiratory distress in the client with an esophageal tamponade is displacement of the esophageal balloon. Before removing the tube, the nurse should deflate both the gastric and esophageal balloons. Answers B and C are incorrect because - applying nasal oxygen or head elevation will not relieve airway obstruction. Answer D is incorrect because increasing the pressure in the esophageal balloon would cause more obstruction of the airway.

74. Mechanical ventilation is give to a client with acute respiratory distress syndrome (ARDS). To increase ventilation and perfusion to all areas of the lungs, what should the nurse do?

a. Tell the client to inhale deeply during the inspiratory cycle.
b. Turn the client every hour.
c. Increase the positive end expiratory pressure (PEEP).
d. Administer medication to prevent the client from fighting the ventilator.

Answer B is correct. By turning the client every hour, the nurse can help increase ventilation and perfusion to all areas of the lungs. To keep the client in constant motion, rocking beds can also be utilized. Answer A is incorrect because respirations are controlled by the ventilator for a client with ARDS. The nurse must have a physician's consent to increase the PEEP, therefore answer C is incorrect. Answer D is incorrect because it will fail to increase ventilation and perfusion.

75. The mother of a child with cystic fibrosis is being taught how to do chest percussion. Which of the following should the nurse tell the mother?

a. Use cupped hands during percussion.
b. Use the heel of her hand during percussion.
c. Change the child's position every 20 minutes during percussion sessions.
d. Do percussion after the child eats and at bedtime.

Answer A is correct. When performing chest percussion, the nurse or parent should use a cupped hand. Answer B is incorrect because the hand needs to be cupped. Answer C is incorrect because the child's position needs to be changed regularly every 5–10 minutes - the session should be restricted to 20 minutes. Chest percussion should be done before meals, therefore answer D is incorrect.

76. Cystic fibrosis is an exocrine disorder that impacts a number systems of the body. Which of the following is the earliest sign associated with cystic fibrosis diagnosis:

a. Steatorrhea
b. Frequent respiratory infections
c. Meconium ileus
d. Increased sweating

Answer C is correct. The earliest sign of cystic fibrosis is meconium ileus, which can be present in a baby with the disease. Answers A, B, and D are incorrect because they are later manifestations.

77. Which of the following is a suggested diet for a child with cystic fibrosis?

a. High calories, high protein, moderate fat
b. High calories, moderate protein, low fat
c. Moderate calories, moderate protein, moderate fat
d. Low calories, high protein, low fat

Answer A is correct. The child with cystic fibrosis requires a diet that is high in calories, with high levels of protein and moderate fat. Answers B, C, and D do not fill the nutritional requirements inflicted by the disease, therefore they are incorrect.

78. Mechanical ventilation with hyperventilation is provided for a client with increased intracranial pressure. Which of the following is the purpose of the hyperventilation:

a. Prevent the development of acute respiratory failure
b. Increase systemic tissue perfusion
c. Prevent cerebral anoxia
d. Decrease cerebral blood flow

Answer D is correct. Hyperventilation decreases swelling and increases intracranial pressure by reducing cerebral blood flow. Answers A, B, and C are incorrect because they are not related to the situation.

79. A client accidentally pulls out the chest tube. They were admitted two days earlier with a lung resection. Which of the following actions indicates understanding of chest tube management by the nurse:

a. Order a chest x-ray.
b. Cover the insertion site with a Vaseline gauze.
c. Reinsert the tube.
d. Call the doctor.

Answer B is correct. The action that the nurse takes first should be to cover the insertion site with an occlusive dressing if the client pulls the chest tube out. The nurse should inform the doctor following this - they will order a chest x-ray and reinsert the tube if needed.
Answers A, C, and D are incorrect because these should not be the first actions to be taken.

80. A mother has cystic fibrosis, and she hopes that her son's children wont have the disease. What should the nurse be aware of?

a. Most of the males with cystic fibrosis are sterile.
b. There is a 25% chance that his children will have cystic fibrosis.
c. There is a 50% chance that his children will be carriers.
d. Most males with cystic fibrosis are capable of having children, so genetic counseling is advised.

Answer A is correct. Due to obstruction of the vas deferens, approx. 99% of males with cystic fibrosis are sterile. Most males with cystic fibrosis are unable to reproduce, therefore answers B, C, and D are incorrect.

81. A client is admitted that is suspected to have Legionnaires' disease. Which of the factors elevates the risk of Legionnaires' disease development?

a. Foreign travel
b. Treatment of arthritis with steroids
c. Eating fresh shellfish twice a week
d. Doing volunteer work at the local hospital

Answer B is correct. Immunosuppression, alcoholism, advanced age, and pulmonary disease are all factors associated with the development of Legionnaires' disease. Answer A is incorrect because it is linked with the SARS development. Answer C is not linked Legionnaires' disease, but with food-borne illness. Answer D is not relevant to this question.

82. **When using a respiratory inhaler, a client asks the nurse to explain how they can find out when half the medication is empty so that they can refill their prescription. Which of the following should the nurse should tell the client to do:**

a. Drop the inhaler in water to see if it floats.
b. Shake the inhaler and listen for the contents.
c. Check for a hissing sound as the inhaler is used.
d. Press the inhaler and watch for the mist.

Answer A is correct. To check the inhaler, the client can drop it into a container of water. When the inhaler is half full, it will float upside down with one-quarter of the container remaining above the line of the water. Answers B, C, and D are incorrect as they do not help determine the level of medication remaining.

83. **In an initial assessment of a newborn, a chest circumference of 34cm and an abdominal circumference of 31cm is measured. Breath sounds are diminished on the left side and the chest is asymmetrical. What should the nurse give priority to?**

a. Providing supplemental oxygen by a ventilated mask
b. Performing auscultation of the abdomen for the presence of active bowel sounds
c. Positioning on the left side with head and chest elevated
d. Inserting a nasogastric tube to check for esophageal patency

Answer C is correct. This assessment indicates that a diaphragmatic hernia is present. The newborn should be positioned on the left side with both their head and chest elevated. This position will allow full inflation of the lung on the right side. Answer A is incorrect because supplemental oxygen for newborns is not given by mask. Answer B is incorrect because bowel sounds are not heard in the abdomen - abdominal contents fill the chest cavity in a baby with diaphragmatic hernia. Answer D is incorrect because Inserting a nasogastric tube to examine for esophageal patency is referring to a baby with esophageal atresia.

84. A client with chest tubes is being cared for by the nurse and notes that the Pleuravac's collection chambers are full. Which of the following should the nurse should:

a. Prepare a new unit for continuing collection.
b. Add more water to the suction-control chamber.
c. Remove the drainage using a 60mL syringe.
d. Milk the tubing to facilitate drainage.

Answer A is correct. The nurse should prepare a new unit for continuing the collection in a situation where the Pleuravac collection chambers are full. Answer B is incorrect because the unit is giving suction, therefore the water amount does not need to be increased. The drainage is not to be removed using a syringe, therefore answer C is incorrect. Answer D is incorrect because milking a chest tube requires a doctor's consent and it is unnecessary in this case.

85. An 18-month-old with acute laryngotracheobronchitis is admitted to the hospital. What should the nurse expect to find when assessing the respiratory status:

a. Strident cough and drooling
b. Inspiratory stridor and harsh cough
c. Wheezing and intercostal retractions
d. Expiratory wheezing and nonproductive cough

Answer B is correct. Laryngotracheobronchitis produces inspiratory stridor and a harsh cough. Answer A is incorrect because this refers to the child with epiglotttis. Answer C is incorrect because this refers to an infant with bronchiolitis. Answer D is incorrect as this refers to an infant with asthma.

86. Aerosol treatments, chest percussion, and postural drainage are ordered for a client with cystic fibrosis. The nurse recognizes that the combination of therapies is to:

a. Decrease respiratory effort and mucous production
b. Increase efficiency of the diaphragm and gas exchange
c. Stimulate coughing and oxygen consumption
d. Dilate the bronchioles and help remove secretions

Answer D is correct. Using aerosol treatments and chest percussion and postural drainage has the objective of dilating the bronchioles and assist with loosening secretions. Answers A, B, and C are incorrect because they are inaccurate.

87. Respiratory distress syndrome (RDS) is diagnosed for a newborn. Which of the following positions is best for maintaining an open airway?

a. Supine, with his neck slightly extended.
b. Prone, with his head turned to one side.
c. Side-lying, with a towel beneath his shoulders.
d. Supine, with his neck slightly flexed.

Answer A is correct. A position to help maintain an open airway is placing the infant supine with the neck slightly extended. Answers B, C, and D do not help maintain an open airway, therefore they are incorrect.

88. Vaccination against influenza is recommended for all employees of a local health clinic. Which of the following months is the influenza vaccine generally given in:

a. November
b. December
c. January
d. February

Answer A is correct. The influenza vaccine is usually given in the fall (October and November). Answers B, C, and D are incorrect.

89. A client is diagnosed with tuberculosis and they ask the nurse when they can return to work. What should the nurse tell the client?

a. He can return to work as soon as he feels well enough.
b. He can return to work after a week of being on the medication.
c. He can return to work when he has three negative sputum cultures.
d. He should think about applying for disability because he will no longer be able to work.

Answer C is correct. The client is allowed to return to work when they have had three negative sputum cultures consecutively. Answers A, B, and D are incorrect.

90. Which clients is the most likely to develop acute respiratory distress syndrome?

a. A 20-year-old with fractures of the tibia
b. A 36-year-old who is HIV positive
c. A 32-year-old with barbiturate overdose
d. A 40-year-old with duodenal ulcers

Answer C is correct. Acute respiratory distress syndrome is commonly caused by drug overdose. Answers A, B, and D are incorrect because they are not linked with the generation of acute respiratory distress syndrome.

91. To determine whether a person has been exposed to tuberculosis, the Mantoux text is used. What will the nurse find if the test is positive?

a. Fluid-filled vesicle
b. Sharply demarcated erythema
c. Circular blanched area
d. Central area of induration

Answer D is correct. The presence of induration indicates a positive Mantoux test. Answers A, B, and C are incorrect because they do not indicate a positive Mantoux test.

92. A client that has had a bronchoscopy has returned. What should the nurse assess before offering the client sips of water?

a. Gag reflex
b. Blood pressure
c. Pupilary response
d. Pulse rate

Answer A is correct. Prior to offering sips of water or other fluids, the nurse should ensure that the gag reflex of the client is intact - this reduces the risk of aspiration. Answers B and D are incorrect because although the should be assessed, they are not relevant to the question. Answer C is not relevant to the question.

93. A quantitative sweat test is scheduled for a child suspected of having cystic fibrosis. Which of the following will be used to analyze the quantitative sweat test:

a. Choloride iontophoresis
b. Pilocarpine iontophoresis
c. Sodium iontophoresis
d. Potassium iontophoresis

Answer B is correct. Pilocarpine is a substance that stimulates sweating, and it is used for cystic fibrosis diagnosis. Answers A and C are incorrect because although chloride and sodium levels in the sweat are measured, they do not stimulate sweating. Answer D is incorrect because it is not related to cystic fibrosis.

94. A COPD client is in respiratory failure. Which results would be the most sensitive indicator to suggest that the client needs a mechanical ventilator?

a. PH 7.23
b. PCO2 58
c. SaO2 90
d. HCO3 30

Answer A is correct. The pH is an correct indicator of acute ventilatory failure and whether a client requires mechanical ventilation. Answer B is incorrect because an elevated PCO2 is not an adequate indictor for administering ventilator support. Answer C is incorrect because an oxygen saturation of 90 would be fairly normal for a client with COPD. Answer D is a standard result.

95. Clients on a respiratory unit are being cared for by the nurse. Which client should be seen first upon receiving the following client reports?

a. Client with emphysema expecting discharge
b. Bronchitis client receiving IV antibiotics
c. COPD client with abnormal PO2
d. Bronchitis client with edema and neck vein distention

Answer D is correct. This client is exhibiting symptoms of heart failure - these symptoms are common in clients with a COPD. Answer A is incorrect because the client is being discharged. Answer C is incorrect because a client with an abnormal PO2 would not be cause for major concern in a client with COPD. Answer B is incorrect because the client.

97. A client upon arrival to the emergency department is being assessed by the nurse. Obstruction of the partial airway is suspected. Which of the following clinical manifestations is a late sign of obstruction of the airway?

a. Cyanotic ear lobes
b. Rales in lungs
c. Restless behavior
d. Inspiratory stridor

Answer A is correct. As the obstruction gets worse, cyanosis and loss of consciousness will occur. Answers C and D are incorrect because they are early symptoms of airway obstruction. Answer B is not a specific clinical manifestation of airway obstruction.

96. The intensive care unit is full. The emergency room called in a report on a client who is ventilator-dependent and is being admitted to the medical surgical unit. What piece of equipment would be essential for the nurse to have at the client's bedside?

a. Cardiac monitor
b. Intravenous controller
c. Oxygen by nasal cannula
d. Manual

Answer D is correct. The manual resuscitator is an essential piece of equipment. Ventilator clients should always have another way of ventilation in case a problem arises. Answers A and B are incorrect, they will not be needed as much as answer D. Answer C is inappropriate for a ventilator client.

97. A client on a ventilator that is set on intermittent mandatory ventilation (IMV) is being cared for. Assessment is eight breaths per minute on the ventilator in IMV mode. The client's respiratory rate is assessed at 13 per minute. Which of the following do these findings indicate?

a. The client is breathing five additional breaths on his own.
b. The client is "fighting" the ventilator and needs medication.
c. Pressure support ventilation is being used.

d. Additional breaths are being delivered by the ventilator.

Answer A is correct. The client is breathing five breaths on their own (subtract 8 from 13). Answers B, C, and D represent incorrect information.

98. Which statement by the client would indicate effective teaching of pursed lipped breathing by the nurse?

a. "I should inhale through my mouth very deeply."
b. "I should tighten my abdominal muscles with inhalation."
c. "I should make inhalation twice as long as exhalation."
d. "I should contract my abdominal muscles with exhalation."

Answer D is correct. The proper technique for pursed lipped breathing is contracting the abdominal muscles with exhalation. Answers A, B, and C are incorrect techniques.

99. The nurse is monitoring the arterial blood gases (ABG) of a client with chest trauma. the results are pH 7.35, PO2 85, PCO2 55, and HCO3 27. Which of the following do these values indicate?

a. Uncompensated respiratory acidosis
b. Uncompensated metabolic acidosis
c. Compensated metabolic acidosis
d. Compensated respiratory acidosis

Answer D is correct. Readings of pH 7.35, PO2 85, PCO2 55, and HCO3 27 demonstrate compensated respiratory acidosis with elevated PCO2 (normal 35–45), low pH of less than 7.4 (normal 7.35–7.45), and high HCO3 with compensation (normal 22–26). Answers A, B, and C are not reflected in the blood gas results listed in the question.

100. A client with lung cancer is receiving a pneumonectomy. Which would likely be excluded from the client's plan of care?

a. Pain-control measures
b. Closed chest drainage
c. Supplemental oxygen administration
d. Coughing and deep-breathing exercises

Answer B is correct. Closed chest drainage causes serous fluid to accumulate in the space to prevent mediastinal shift, therefore it is generally not usually used. Answers A, C, and D are all necessary care measures for a lung surgery client.

101. A client following a crushing injury to the chest is being cared for by the nurse. Which of the following findings would most indicate a tension pneumothorax?

a. Expectoration of moderate amounts of frothy hemoptysis
b. Subcutaneous emphysema noted at the anterior chest
c. Trachea shift toward the unaffected side of the chest
d. Opening chest wound with a whistle sound emitting from the area

Answer C is correct. Trachea shift distinguishes this clinical manifestation as a tension pneumothorax. Air enters but cannot escape when a person has a tension pneumothorax. This causes a buildup of pressure and shifting of the great vessels, the trachea, and the heart to the unaffected side. Answer A is incorrect because it is associated with a pulmonary contusion. Answers B and D are incorrect because they are associated with a pneumothorax, but not a tension pneumothorax.

Gastrointestinal Disorders

Section 1: Introduction to Gastrointestinal Disorders

The gastrointestinal system (GI system) is roughly 25 feet long in an adult. The GI tract is made up of the esophagus, gallbladder, liver, mouth, pancreas, salivary glands, small and large intestine, and the stomach.

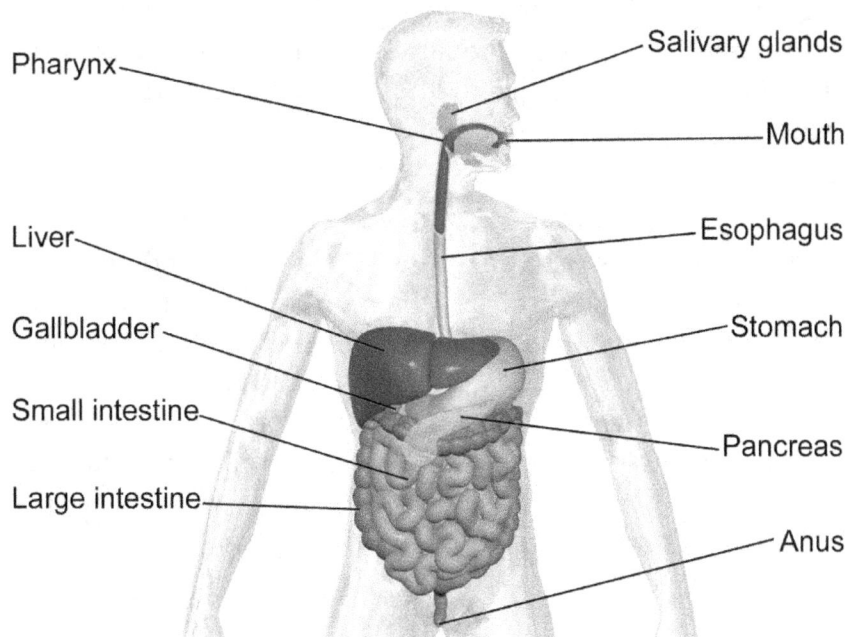

The main functions of the GI system include the digestion and absorption of nutrients, and the elimination of waste products. Gastrointestinal disorders can lead to impaired organ function, problems relating to nutrient extraction, and problems relating to waste elimination. Such complications can be acute, chronic, and life-threatening. On top of this, other problems such as cancer and infection can also occur.

For future nurses, having a very good understanding of the various diseases of the gastrointestinal and digestive system is important in order to provide appropriate care to patients. The NCLEX exam will test your knowledge of gastrointestinal disorders and procedures and it is therefore crucial to really come to grips with this topic and to spend enough time reviewing the care of clients gastrointestinal and digestive disorders. On top of this, it is also crucial to practice applying your knowledge with multiple practice questions. This concise preparation guide will cover the key points that you will need to know to be successful in the respiratory portion of your NCLEX test.

The guide begins with an outline of the topics and key facts on gastrointestinal disorders that you need to remember for the exam. The list of subtopics can be seen on the contents page. In Section 3 of this guide you can apply and test your knowledge with over 100 topic-specific practice questions. All answers to the questions are given, along with detailed rationales for correct and incorrect answers to further your knowledge and understanding of the topic.

Remember that ambition is the first step to success. The second step is action – hard work and determination. Purchasing this guide is an indication of your ambition, now it's time to get to work!

Best wishes,

Eva Regan

Section 2: Gastrointestinal Disorders Study Checklist

In this section, we will firstly cover the major anatomic structures of the GI system before touching upon the key terms and diagnostic exams the nurse and nursing student should be aware of when caring for clients with GI disorders. We will then go on to cover the various diseases that the NCLEX candidate should be familiar with, their causes, symptoms, as well as the appropriate nursing interventions and procedures.

1. <u>Key terms and concepts</u>

Before we talk about the key terms and diagnosis exams the nurse and test-taker should be familiar with, it is firstly important to start with the structure of the GI system. The illustration below shows the GI system's major anatomic structures. Knowing these structures will not only help you conduct accurate client assessments, but will also facilitate your understanding in relation to how the system works and how the different organs interact.

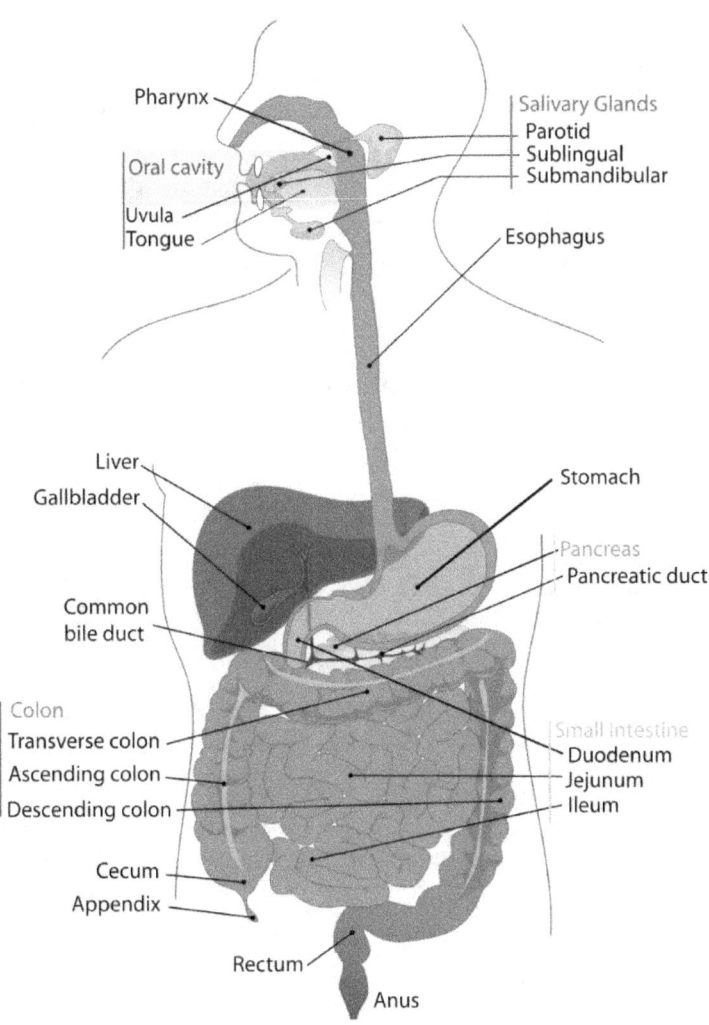

On top of having a sound understanding the anatomic structures of the GI system, you will also need remember and have a good understanding of the following key terms:

- **Ascites:** Ascites refers to the abnormal accumulation of more than 25ml of fluid in the peritoneal cavity which causes abdominal swelling.

- **Gastrinoma:** Gastrinoma is a gastrin-excreting tumor which can occur in the pancreas or in the duodenum. Gastrin is the hormone which controls the amount of acid in the stomach. Large amounts of gastrin cause the stomach to make more acid which in turn leads to the formation of ulcers in the stomach and small bowel.

- **Hepatomegaly:** Hepatomegaly is the abnormal enlargement of the liver.

- **Melena:** Melena is the passage of stools that appear dark or tarry. It is an indication of bleeding in the esophagus, stomach, or the first part part of the small intestine.

- **Odynophagia:** Odynophagia is a term for painful swallowing. The pain may stem from the esophagus or the mouth.

- **Splenomegaly:** Splenomegaly is the abnormal enlargement of the spleen.

- **Steatorrhea:** Steatorrhea is the presence of excess fats in stools. Fatty stool is oily, bulky, malodorous and often float on top of the toilet water. It is caused by reduced absorption of fat by the intestines.

- **Tetany:** Tetany is a condition characterized by the involuntary contraction of muscles.

Besides the usual routine examinations, the nurse should also be aware and have an understanding of the following diagnostic exams which form an integral part of nursing care for clients with gastrointestinal disorders:

- Barium enema
- Barium swallow
- Colonoscopy and sigmoidoscopy
- Endoscopic exams
- Gallbladder ultrasound
- Gastric analysis and biopsy
- H. Pylori
- Liver biopsy
- Liver panel blood tests
- pH motility studies
- Upper GI studies

2. <u>Appendicitis</u>

The appendix is located in the right lower abdomen and is attached to the cecum. Appendicitis is most common in adolescents and males are more prone to infections of the appendix than females.

Symptoms of appendicitis include:

- Epigastric or periumbilical pain in the right lower quadrant of the abdomen (the Mcburney's point). A positive Rovsing's sign can also occur.
- Low-grade fewer

- Nausea
- Vomiting

Diagnosis:

- Laboratory findings reveal an elevated white blood cell count and neutrophil count (a left shift).
- CT scan shows right lower quadrant denseness with bowel distention

Treatment:

- To Treat clients with appendicitis, an appendectomy is required to remove the infected and inflamed appendix.

Nursing intervention:

- Administration of analgesics
- Administration of IV fluids to prevent dehydration
- Administration of antibiotics to treat infection
- A solid food diet after the surgery

Provided surgery was complication-free, the client will usually be discharged the same day or the day after surgery. The nurse and nursing student should also be aware of the fact that enemas and laxatives are contraindicated and can lead to perforation in clients with appendicitis.

3. <u>Cholecystitis/Cholelithiasis</u>

Cholecystitis is inflammation of the gallbladder. Cholelithiasis, or gallstone disease, involves the presence of one or more gallstones in the gallbladder. Gallstones form when bile which is usually stored in the gallbladder solidifies and hardens to form stones. Gallstones are composed mainly of cholesterol, bilirubin, and calcium.

The following factors can increase a person's risk of developing gallbladder problems:

- A family history of gallbladder problems
- Being female and above the age of forty
- Crohn's disease
- Diabetes
- Dietary habits (being overweight or obese)
- Haemolytic blood disorders
- Use of certain medications, e.g. cholesterol-lowering agents

Symptoms of Cholecystitis include:

- Pain
- Jaundice of the skin
- Sclerae
- Upper palate

Symptoms of Cholelithiasis include:

- Abdominal distention
- Abdominal pain in the right upper quadrant
- Abdominal pain which radiates to the right shoulder
- Dark urine
- Dyspepsia
- Fever
- Flatulence
- Nausea
- Steatorrhea
- Stools which are clay-colored
- Vomiting

Diagnosis of Cholecystitis and Cholelithiasis:

- Abdominal x-ray
- ERCP (used in clients with allergies to contrast media)
- Gallbladder ultrasound (routine test for diagnosis)
- Heptobiliary scan

Treatment of Cholecystitis:

Treatment may be conservative or surgical. Conservative treatment of Cholecystitis is achieved by maintaining the client NPO with NG suction and IV fluids. To assist with spasm of the smooth muscles, anticholinergics are administered. If the client's WBC count is elevated, antibiotics are administered intravenously. Once recovery has begun, the client is placed on a high-protein, low-fats liquids, and high-carbohydrate diet.

Foods to encourage:

- Bread
- Coffee and tea
- Cooked fruits
- Flatulence-free vegetables
- Lean meats
- Mashed potatoes
- Rice
- Skim milk
- Tapioca

Foods to avoid:

- Alcohol
- Cheese
- Cream
- Eggs
- Flatulent vegetables
- Fried foods
- Pork
- Rich dressings

Treatment of Cholelithiasis:

Cholelithiasis is treated using surgery, PO medication,

lithotripsy procedures.

- **Ursodeoxycholic acid (UDCA) or chenodeoxycholic acid (CDCA)can be used to treat small stones and radiolucent stones.** These medications are bile acids and can dissolve gallstones. This treatment however can take up to two years and is therefore utilized mostly on clients that are not good surgery candidates, such as elderly clients. Half the clients who are treated in this way experience a recurrence of the stones once the therapy has ended.

- **Extracorporeal shock wave lithotripsy (ESWL) can also be used to treat clients with gallstones.** Shock waves are used to fragments the gallstones which are then expelled from the body through the common bile ducts, dissolved by acid medications, or retrieved by endoscopy.

- **Surgery (laparoscopic or abdominal cholecystectomy) can also be used to remove gallstones.** Laparoscopy surgery is more common and its advantages include quicker resumption of post-op activity, less post-op pain, and a decreased possibility of occurring paralytic ileus. Abdominal surgery removes larger gallstones and is reserved for those with extensive involvement of the duct system.

4. Clostridium Difficile

C. difficile or Clostridium difficile is a bacterial infection that upsets the healthy balance of bacteria in the digestive system and which can cause symptoms ranging from diarrhea to more serious inflammations of the colon which can be life-threatening.

The following factors can increase a person's risk of developing C. difficile:

- Antibiotic therapy
- Being elderly
- Immunosuppressed clients
- Lengthy hospital stays
- Postoperative gastrointestinal surgery

Symptoms of C. difficile include:

- Abdominal cramping
- Abdominal pain
- Fever
- Watery diarrhea

Diagnosis of C. difficile:

- Assessment of stool culture for C. difficile

Treatment of C. difficile:

- Administration of antibiotics (Flagyl or Vancomycin)

- Infection control: this includes placing infected clients in private rooms, hand hygiene, taking contact precautions, and teaching family members accordingly.

5. Liver Diseases

Liver diseases are common and can be the result of a variety of factors and can affect men, women, and children. Liver disease can be hereditary or caused by a variety of factors that damage the liver, such as alcohol or viruses. In this section, we will cover the causes, diagnosis, symptoms, and treatment of the liver failures which candidates will need to know for the NCLEX exam. They include the following: Cirrhosis, Hepatitis A, Hepatitis B, Hepatitis C, Hepatitis D, Hepatitis E, Hepatitis G, and Pancreatitis.

CIRRHOSIS

Cirrhosis is scarring of the liver. Scarring, or fibrosis, can lead to the distortion of the liver structures and vessels.

The most common causes of cirrhosis include:

- Alcoholism
- Hepatitis

Symptoms of cirrhosis include:

- Abnormal enlargement of the liver (hepatomegaly)
- Abnormal enlargement of the spleen (spleenomegaly)
- Ascites, which leads to abdominal swelling
- Behavioural changes and changes in cognition and speech
- Chronic indigestion
- Constipation
- Diarrhea
- Edema
- Increased ammonia levels
- Increased blood urea nitrogen (BUN) levels
- Increased liver enzymes
- Jaundice (yellowed skin)
- Petechiae
- Vitamin A, D, E, and K deficiencies
- Weight loss

Diagnosis tests for cirrhosis:

- CT scan
- Esophagogastroduodenoscopy (EGD)
- Laboratory tests (ammonia levels, liver enzymes, prothrombin time)
- Liver biopsy
- Upper gastrointestinal x-ray

Treatment of cirrhosis:

- Encourage a diet rich in calories, rich in protein, and low in sodium, i.e. a diet which promotes healing of liver tissue – remember: protein sources will be restricted if the client is in end-stage failure
- For injections, use small needles only and maintain pressure for five minutes after injections due to bleeding tendencies
- Heme-test all stools and vomitus
- Instruct the client to avoid alcohol
- Instruct the client to avoid medications detoxified by the liver
- Measure abdominal girth every day
- Monitor intake and output
- Monitor the client's weight
- Prescribe antacids to relieve gastric distress
- Prescribe cathartics and enemas to correct the pH in the bowel and to reduce ammonia in the body
- Prescribe diuretics if the client is retaining fluids and to relieve antacids

HEPATITIS

Hepatitis is a viral infection of the liver. There are five major types of hepatitis: A, B, C, D, and E. Hepatitis A and E are transmitted through contaminated water, food, and human waste. Hepatitis B, C, and D are also similar in that they can be transmitted parenterally, perinatally, or sexually. Lastly, hepatitis G can also be transmitted parenterally, at birth, through blood transfusion and sexual contact.

Whatever the type of hepatitis infection, the nurse should be aware of the following care interventions which apply to all clients with hepatitis. The nurse should:

- Administer medications such as steroids, anti-inflammatory drugs, and immunosuppressives
- Advise clients to avoid medications detoxified by the liver
- Encourage a diet of small and frequent increased calorie meals
- Increase the client's fluid intake to 3000 ml/day
- Keep clients with prodromal or icteric symptoms on bed rest
- Practice standard precaution control measures while providing care
- Treat pruritus with cool baths and soothing lotions

Before discussing the various types of viral hepatitis infections, it is important for nurses and nursing students to know and understand the two stages of hepatitis. Whichever type of hepatitis the client has contracted, the symptoms experienced are associated with two stages: the prodromal stage and the icteric stage.

The prodromal stage is the period of time during which the client is experiencing vague symptoms. During this period, the client will experience abnormal bile secretion – indicated by clay-colored stools and dark urine. The prodromal stage can last anywhere from a few days to two weeks and symptoms include the following:

- Anorexia
- Clay-colored stools
- Dark urine
- Fatigue
- Fever
- Nausea
- Vomiting

The bile slowly accumulates in the client's blood which is when the icteric stage begins and the client starts experiencing other symptoms which include:

- Elevated liver enzymes
- Hepatomegaly
- Jaundice
- Pruritus
- Tenderness in the upper right quadrant of the abdomen

HEPATITIS A

Hepatitis A, a viral liver disease which is transmitted by the fecal-oral route, can cause mild to severe illness. Note that Hepatitis A is not chronic and has no long-term effects.

The symptoms of Hepatitis A which usually appear after a 2-6 incubation period include:

- Fever

- Jaundice
- Malaise
- Nausea
- Vomiting

Diagnosis of Hepatitis A:

- Diagnosis is made by a stool specimen – detection of the Hepatitis A antigen can be made 7-10 days before the illness shows and 2-3 weeks after symptoms appear.

There is no specific treatment for Hepatitis A. Because of this, prevention plays a key role. The following are the most effective ways to combat Hepatitis A. It is important to remember the three medications for the exam.

- **Hepatitis A vaccine (Havrix).** Adults above the age of 18 are encouraged to receive the two-dose hepatitis vaccine. Homosexuals, healthcare workers, and people travelling to unsanitary countries are strongly encouraged to get vaccinated. Once vaccinated, protection lasts for up to 20 years.
- **Hepatitis A and hepatitis B combination drug (Twinrix).** Twinrix can be administered for people aged 18 and older.
- **Serum immune globulin.** The immune globulin should be administered within 2 weeks of exposure to the disease. It serves to boost antibody protection and provides passive immunity for 6-8 weeks.
- **Improved sanitation and food safety.**

HEPATITIS B

Hepatitis B can be transmitted parentally, perinatally, or sexually. After hepatitis B enters the body, there is an incubation period of 1.5 to 6 months. People at greatest risk of obtaining hepatitis B include infants that are born to mothers who are positive for hepatitis B, IV drug users, healthcare workers, hemodialysis clients, and homosexual men.

The symptoms of hepatitis B include:

- Abdominal pain
- Arthritis
- Fever
- Jaundice
- Malaise
- Nausea
- Rash

Diagnosis of Hepatitis B:

- HBsAG, the surface antigen of hepatitis B, can be detected in the blood for 2-8 weeks before symptoms appear and for 2-8 weeks after exposure to the virus.

Prevention and treatment of Hepatitis B:

- **Hepatitis B vaccine (HeptovaxRecombivax).** The vaccine is given in three injections via the intramuscular route into the deltoid muscle. The second doze is given one month after the first dose and the third dose is given after six months.
- **Alpha interferon injections are administered to treat chronic hepatitis B infections.** In the 3 to 6 hours following the administration, the client may exhibit flu-like symptoms. Subcutaneous injections for PEGintron or Pegasys are given once weekly.
- **Hepatitis B immune globin (HBIG).** This immune globin should be administered within 24 hours following exposure to hepatitis B. It is designed to provide passive immunity to people who have been exposed to the HBV but have not received the hepatitis B vaccine.
- **Nucleoside analogs to treat HIV infection.** These are medications that can be administered once yearly and which can be given orally. They include: Adefovir (Hepsera), entecavir (Baraclude), lamivudine (Epivir), and telbivudine (Tyzeka.)

HEPATITIS C

Hepatitis C, like hepatitis B, can be transmitted parentally, perinatally, or sexually. Compared to the other types of viral hepatitis, more people with hepatitis C progress to a chronic carrier state. In one out of four patients with chronic hepatitis C, the liver disease can lead to more serious problems including cirrhosis, liver failure and liver cancer.

Symptoms of Hepatitis C:

- Symptoms are similar to those of hepatitis B although some say that symptoms are variable and mild.
- Chronic hepatitis C is said to be a 'silent' disease because often no symptoms appear. Because of this, infected people rarely seek medical assistance.

Diagnosis of Hepatitis C:

- Diagnosis is confirmed by the presence of HCV, the hepatitis C virus, in the blood serum.
- A liver biopsy may also be performed.

Treatment of Hepatitis C:

- There is no available vaccine for hepatitis C.
- Medications for the treatment of hepatitis C include a combination therapy of alpha interferon and ribavirin.

HEPATITIS D

Hepatitis D is caused by the the hepatitis D virus (HDV) which can only propagate in the presence of the hepatitis B virus (HBV). Because of this, only people with hepatitis B are at risk for hepatitis D. The incubation period 3 to 20 weeks for hepatitis D. HDV infections are most common among IV drug users, hemodialysis clients and those who have received multiple blood transfusions. The symptoms are similar to those of exhibited by clients with hepatitis B, although clients with hepatitis D are more likely to develop cirrhosis and more prone to developing chronic hepatitis.

Diagnosis of Hepatitis D:

- Diagnosis of hepatitis D is made by a lab test which will reveal the presence of anti-delta bodies in the presence of the hepatitis B antigen (HBAg).

Treatment of Hepatitis D:

- Treatment includes the alpha interferon, which may be administered for up to 12 months for a long-term HDV infection.

HEPATITIS E

Hepatitis E, like hepatitis A, is transmitted by the fecal-oral route and is also not chronic. Symptoms for hepatitis E are similar to experienced by clients with hepatitis A. The incubation period for this hepatitis is 15 to 54 days.

Diagnosis of Hepatitis E:

- Diagnosis is confirmed by the presence of anti-HEV (hepatitis E virus) in the blood serum.

Treatment of Hepatitis E:

- There is no available treatment for hepatitis E. Post-exposure treatment with immune globin has not shown to be effective.
- Preventative measures should be taken through the practice of good hygiene and hand-washing.

HEPATITIS G

Hepatitis G is caused by the hepatitis G virus (HGV) which is transmitted parenterally, sexually, and by blood transfusions. There is currently no treatment for hepatitis G.

PANCREATITIS

Pancreatitis is the inflammation of the pancreas. Pancreatic damage happens when digestive enzymes are activated before they are released into the small intestine and start destroying the tissue of the pancreas.

The following are some factors which can cause Pancreatitis:

- Alcoholism (long-term and heavy alcohol use is a common contributing cause in middle-aged men with pancreatitis)
- Bacterial or viral infections
- Biliary disease
- Blunt abdominal trauma
- Endoscopic retrograde cholangiopancreatography (ERCP) procedure
- Ischemic vascular disease
- Long-term use of oral contraceptives, opiates, steroids, thiazide diuretics, oral contraceptives, or sulfonamides
- Peptic ulcer disease
- Surgery on or near the pancreas

Symptoms of Pancreatitis include:

- Abdominal distention
- Decreased calcium levels
- Elevated amylase levels
- Elevated blood and urine glucose levels
- Elevated lipase levels
- Elevated white blood cells counts
- Epigastric pain radiating to the back
- Nausea

- Steatorrhea (fatty stools)
- Vomiting

Diagnosis of Pancreatitis:

- Lab tests revealing elevated white blood cell counts, elevated glucose levels, and elevated serum lipase and amylase levels
- Lab tests revealing decreased serum calcium levels
- Endoscopic retrograde cholangiopancreatography (ERCP) (if gallstones are causing pancreatitis)
- CT scans
- MRI scans

Treatment of Pancreatitis:

- For acute pancreatitis, clients are kept NPO and will receive IV fluids to maintain blood pressure and to replace lost fluids.
- Clients should also be monitored for signs of bleeding. To prevent excessive bleeding, small-gauge needles should be used for any injections and pressure should be maintained for five minutes after the the injection has been given.
- Once oral feedings begin, the diet should be low-fat and low-protein and both alcohol and caffeine should be avoided.
- ABGs should be monitored to detect any early complications.
- Surgery may be required if ERCP doesn't remove all gallstones or if there are other complications such as

abscess formation or pancreatic pseudocyst (collection of fluid around the pancreas).

Medications to treat pancreatitis include:

- Antibiotics
- Calcium gluconate
- Histamine 2 blockers
- Insulin
- Narcotic analgesics
- Viokase
- Vitamins A, D, E, and K

6. Diverticulitis

Diverticulosis is the condition which occurs with the presence of presence of diverticula (sac-like outpouchings) in the wall of the large intestine. Diverticulitis is the inflammation of the diverticulum, especially in the colon, which increases the risk of perforation and abscess formation. Diverticulitis is caused by the trapping of bacteria and food in the diverticula. It is most common in elderly females with a diet rich in nuts, grains, and seeds.

Symptoms of Diverticulitis include:

- Bowel irregularity
- Cramping pain in the lower left quadrant of the abdomen

- Low-grade fever
- Spells of diarrhea

Diagnosis of Diverticulitis:

- A complete blood count (CBC) which can reveal an elevation in white blood cells due to the infection and an elevation in sedimentation rate that indicates inflammation.
- CT scan to determine whether an abscess has formed.
- Barium enema studies to demonstrate diverticulitis with thickening of the muscle and the narrowing of the colon – **note however that** a barium studies can be contraindicated in clients with acute diverticulitis because of the potential of perforation of the diverticulum.
- Endoscopy exam to detect the inflamed diverticulum.

Treatment of Diverticulitis:

- Increase diet intake of soft fiber foods – **note however that** a low fiber diet is encouraged during the acute episode
- Increase in fluid intake of around 2–3 liters per day within cardiac limits
- Administrate medications such as analgesics, antibiotics, antispasmodics, and fiber laxatives
- Surgery may be required if the client's symptoms don't improve with conservative therapy (diet alterations and administration of medications). Surgery may also be necessary in the case of abscess

formation, bowel obstruction, hemorrhage, or perforation

7. Food-Borne Illnesses

Food-borne illness occur when a person ingests an infectious organism. Food-borne illnesses often cause gastrointestinal problems. It is important to remember the most common types of illnesses, their causes and symptoms, as listed below.

Botulism

Incubation period:
- 18-36 hours

Causes:
- Improperly canned vegetables and fruit
- Occasionally meats and fish

Preventative measures:
- Canning containers should be boiled for at least 20 minutes
- Meat should be cooked thoroughly

Symptoms:
- Diarrhea
- Dysarthria
- Dysphagia
- Nausea

- Paralysis
- Respiratory failure
- Vomiting
- Weakness

Treatment:
- Antitoxin
- IV fluid replacement
- NPO
- Respiratory support
- Trivalent botulism

E. coli

Incubation period:
- Varies depending on the strain of E. coli

Causes:
- Food contaminated with feces
- Undercooked beef and shellfish

Preventative measures:
- Meat should be cooked thoroughly

Symptoms:
- Abdominal cramping
- Diarrhea
- Fever
- Vomiting
- Potentially life-threatening if organ failure and rapid fluid loss occurs

Treatment:

- Administration of antibiotics
- IV fluid replacement

Salmonella

Incubation period:
- 8-24 hours

Causes:
- Contaminated food and fluids
- Raw eggs

Preventative measures:
- Hand-washing

Symptoms:
- Abdominal pain
- Cramping
- Diarrhea
- Fever
- Nausea
- Vomiting

Treatment:
- IV fluid administration
- NPO

Staphylococcal

Incubation period:
- 2-4 hours

Causes:
- Can be transmitted via a human carrier
- Meat
- Milk and dairy products

Preventative measures:
- Store and prepare food properly

Symptoms:
- Abdominal cramping
- Diarrhea
- Sudden vomiting
- Weakness

Treatment:
- Replacement of electrolytes
- Replacement of lost fluid volume

8. <u>Gastroesophageal reflux disease (GERD)</u>

GERD, which stands for gastroesophageal reflux disease, is an esophageal disorder which occurs when there is a complication which allows contents to reflux back into the esophagus. Hiatal hernia occurs when the stomach pushes up through the diaphragm. Long-term reflux can lead to Barrett's esophagus, which is a serious complication of GERD which can lead to esophageal cancer.

The symptoms of GERD include:

- Chest pain
- Dyspepsia
- Dysphagia
- Eructation
- Painful swallowing (dynophagia)

Diagnosis of GERD:

- Monitoring the pH
- Endoscopic exam
- Esophagram or Barium swallow

Treatment of GERD:

- Administration of medications, including antacids, histamine blockers, and proton pump inhibitors
- Avoidance of alcohol and carbonated beverages
- Avoidance of irritating foods, such as acidic foods, chocolate, and fats
- Diet with frequent small meals
- Endoscopic procedure: Stretta
- Instruct client to remain upright for 2–3 hours after eating
  Avoidance of eating within three hours of bedtime
- Surgery: Laparoscopic Nissen fundoplication (LNF)
- Treatment for Barrett's esophagus is by way of periodic exams to detect and treat precancerous cells in order to avoid esophageal cancer.

9. Hemorrhoids

Hemorrhoids are swollen vein(s) in the anal area which are caused by anything which increases pressure in the anal area, such as pregnancy or constipation. Hemorrhoids are classified as **internal** if located above the anal sphincter. Hemorrhoids are classified as **external** if located outside the anal sphincter.

Symptoms of Hemorrhoids include:

- Blood in stools
- Itching in the anal area
- Pain in the anal area

Treatment of Hemorrhoids is focused on relieving the symptoms and include:

- Astringent pads
- Cold packs
- Increase fluids and fiber in diet
- Local pain-relieving ointments/suppositories
- Rest
- Sitz baths
- Warm compresses
- Surgery (hemorrhoidectomy) may be required if the client is experiencing advanced thrombosis of the vein
- For non-thrombotic hemorrhoid, infrared photocoagulation and rubber band ligation can also be used for treatment

10. Inflammatory Bowel Disease

Inflammatory bowel disorders are most common in people aged 10-30. The causes are not known but the disorders can be triggered by food additives, pesticides, and radiation. There are two major types of inflammatory bowel disease: Crohn's disease and ulcerative colitis.

CROHN'S DISEASE (REGIONAL ENTERITIS)

Crohn's disease is a chronic inflammatory disease of the intestines, which can result in abscess formation, swelling and thickening.

The symptoms of Crohn's disease include:

- Abdominal pain
- Anemia
- Cramping
- Diarrhea
- Ulcer formation
- Weight loss

Diagnosis of Crohn's disease:

- Barium studies which reveal a positive string sign – a string sign is the narrowing of the lumen of the intestine

Treatment of Crohn's disease:

- Encourage a low-residue diet
- Medications, including antidiarrheals, antirheumatics, immunosuppressives, sedatives, and steroids
- Surgery (colectomy with possible ileostomy) for severe cases
- Vitamin and iron supplements

ULCERATIVE COLITIS

Ulcerative colitis is the inflammation of the colon and the rectum. This disease can cause long-lasting inflammation and ulcers and can cause systematic complications and a high mortality rate.

The symptoms of Ulcerative Colitis include:

- Abdominal cramping
- Bloody diarrhea
- Decreased iron absorption
- Fever
- Urgent defecation
- Vomiting
- Weight loss

Diagnosis of Ulcerative Colitis:

- Barium enema
- Sigmoidoscopy

Treatment of Ulcerative Colitis;

- Treatment of ulcerative colitis is similar to that of Crohn's disease
- Additional drugs which may be administered to treat ulcerative colitis include: antibiotics and anti-inflammatories

11. Intestinal Obstructions

Intestinal obstruction is the blockage that keeps food or liquid from passing through the intestinal tract. Intestinal obstructions can be **functional** – because of the lack of adequate muscle to propel contents through the small or large intestine, e.g. due to muscular dystrophy – **or mechanical** – caused by pressure on the wall of the intestine, e.g. due to a tumor.

Small intestine bowel obstructions are more frequent and are commonly caused by adhesions. Large bowel obstructions often occur in the sigmoid colon. Common causes of intestinal obstruction include carcinomas and hernias.

Symptoms of Small Bowel Obstruction include:

- Abdominal distention in the upper abdomen
- Colicky abdominal pain
- Inability to have a bowel movement
- Nausea
- Vomiting

Symptoms of Large Bowel Obstruction include:

- Abdominal distention in the lower abdomen
- Inability to have a bowel movement or thin and loose stool
- Pain which is usually located lower abdomen
- Some vomiting

Diagnosis of Intestinal Obstruction:

- Assessment of abdominal blood gas (metabolic alkalosis will indicate small bowel obstruction and metabolic acidosis will indicate large bowel obstruction)
- CT scan to assess cause of the intestinal obstruction
- Flat and upright abdominal X-rays

Treatment of Intestinal Obstruction:

- Administer pain medication (remember here that pain medication may be withheld at initial stages to determine the client's problem)
- Assess NG tube for patency
- Assess urinary output, skin turgor, and mucous membranes to monitor fluids
- Monitor electrolytes in blood serum

- Monitor IV fluid replacement therapy
- Monitor the abdominal girth daily
- Monitor the client for nausea, emesis, and increasing abdominal distention
- Monitor vital signs for abnormalities
- Surgery (exploratory laparotomy) may be performed to determine and correct the cause of the obstruction

12. Peritonitis

Peritonitis is the inflammation of the peritoneum. Common causes include bacterial infection either via the blood or after rupture of an abdominal organ, appendicitis, diverticulitis, and perforated ulcer.

The symptoms of Peritonitis include:

- Abdominal tenderness
- Pain and increase pain with movement
- Rebound tenderness
- Rigidity of the abdomen
- Signs of paralytic ileus, such as abdominal distention and absent bowel signs

Diagnosis of Peritonitis:

- Abdominal X-rays which reveal air and fluid with a swollen/bloated bowel.
- CBC lab exam which reveals an elevated WBC, decreased hematocrit, and decreased hemoglobin.
- CT scan which shows abscess formation.

Treatment of Peritonitis:

- Administration of IV antibiotics to prevent and treat infection
- Administration of IV fluid
- Administration of nausea medication
- Administration of pain medication
- Monitor client's intake and output
- Monitor for complications (e.g. abscess formation and wound dehiscence or evisceration)
- Monitor IV fluid intake
- Oxygen administration (because fluid in the abdomen can cause respiratory difficulties)
- Placement of an NG tube to relieve abdominal distention
- Surgical intervention to remove the cause of the peritonitis
- If the client reports feelings of something 'bursting open', it is important to immediately assess the client's wound and to report findings to the doctor. If wound dehiscence occurs, the nurse should apply a non-adherent or moist saline dressing and notify the surgeon.

13. Ulcers

Ulcers are open sores that occur in the mucosal lining of the esophagus, duodenum, or stomach. Men, post-menopausal women, those with type O blood, and those with a family history of ulcers are most prone to ulcers.

Causes which contribute to the development of ulcers include:

- Infection with *H. Pylori* bacteria
- Irritants that promote elevated secretion of hydrochloric acid
- Non-steroidal anti-inflammatory drugs (NSAIDs), e.g. toradol and ibuprofen
- Steroids
- It is important to remember that NSAIDS and steroids should be administered with food
- Stress

Ulcers can be esophageal, duodenal, or gastric depending on where the ulcer is located in the GI system. Duodenum and gastric ulcers are the most common.

Duodenal ulcers, which are most common in people aged 30 to 50, are open sores that are located on the mucosa of the duodenum. Symptoms and signs of duodenal ulcers include:

- Epigastric pain which occurs 2-3 hours after food intake
- Melena
- Pain which Is relieved by eating
- Vomiting is very uncommon with duodenal ulcers

Gastric ulcers, which are most common in people above the age of 50, are open sores located in the gastric mucosa. Symptoms and signs of gastric ulcers include:

- Discomfort which is aggravated by food intake

- Midepigastric pain which occurs from 30-60 minutes after food intake
- Vomiting

Diagnosis of Ulcers:

- Assessment of the client's history
- Biopsy
- Detection of H. Pylori bacteria which can be done via a blood test, stool exam, or C13 urea breath test
- Endoscopy exam
- Esophagram or barium swallow
- Gastric analysis
- Upper gastrointestinal (GI) studies

Treatment of Ulcers:

- Administration of medications, such as
  o Antacids
  o Antibiotics
  o Anticholinergics
  o Antispasmodics
  o Barrier drugs such sucralfate (Carafate)
  o Histamine blockers
  o Prostandin analogues such as misoprostol (Cytotec)
  o Proton pump inhibitors
- Avoiding alcohol
- Avoiding seasoned or spicy food
- Avoiding smoking
- Encouraging a diet high in fiber foods
- Reducing stress
- Surgery (gastrectomy) may also be performed. Post-op care includes assessment of abdominal distention,

bleeding, and shock. After gastrectomy, the NG tube should not be moved or irrigated without a specific order by the doctor.

DUMPING SYNDROME

This is a complication which may arise in clients who have undergone gastric surgery. It is a group of symptoms that can be caused by the rapid removal of food from the stomach into the jejunum.

Symptoms of Dumping Syndrome include:

- Dizziness
- Nausea
- Pallor
- Palpitations
- Vomiting

Treatment of Dumping Syndrome include:

- Administering medications, such as
  - Antispasmodics and sedatives such as bentyl and pro-banthine
  - Somastatin analogues such as octreotide (sandostatin)
- Advising the client to remain in recumbent position after meals
- Decreasing carbohydrate intake
- Decreasing fluids that are given with meals

- Providing small and frequent meals

Irritable Bowel Syndrome (IBS)

IBS is a common disorder that affects the large intestine and is characterized by irregular bowel patterns. IBS can be classified as IBS constipation, IBS diarrhea, or IBS mixed constipation and diarrhea. The cause of IBS is unknown although it is thought that anxiety, depression, hormones, gastroenteritis, stress, and certain types of food are contributing factors.

Symptoms of Irritable Bowel Syndrome include:

- A feeling of incomplete evacuation of stool
- Abdominal pain
- Bloating
- Constipation
- Diarrhea
- Excessive accumulation of gas

Diagnosis of Irritable Bowel Syndrome:

- Diagnosis can be made by ruling out other diseases that may cause the symptoms, such as ulcer disease or colorectal cancer
- Assessment of the client's history
- Physical exam
- Sigmoidoscopy which can reveal pain and spastic contractions

Treatment of Irritable Bowel Syndrome:

- Administering medications, such as
  - Alosetron (Lotrenox) for diarrhea.
  - Anti-spasmodics, e.g. dicyclomine (Bentyl) for abdominal pain
  - Loperamide (Imodium)
- Avoiding of gas-causing foods such as apple juice, grapes, milk, and sugarless gum
- Hypnosis and acupuncture can also be used as complementary therapies
- Reducing stress

14. Pharmacological Interventions to Treat Gastrointestinal Disorders

Pharmacological interventions play a central role in caring for clients with GI disorders. It is important for the NCLEX test-taker to remember and have a good understanding of the medications commonly administered to treat, improve, or cure disorders of the GI system. The nurse and nursing student will also need to know the drug classification and the common side and adverse effects of the drug.

Below we have included some of the most commonly used agents, their actions, side effects, and the relevant nursing intervention that is required.

Esomeprazole (Nexium) – proton pump inhibitor

- **Action:**
  - Decreases acid

- **Side effects:**
  - o Abdominal pain
  - o Diarrhea
  - o Headache
  - o Increased blood sugar
  - o Intestinal gas
- **Nursing intervention:**
  - o Chew pellets should not be crushed
  - o Capsules can be emptied into a tablespoon of applesauce to be swallowed immediately
  - o Monitor the client for hememsesis
  - o Monitor the client for melena

Famotidine (Pepcid) – H2 antagonist

- **Action:**
  - o Manages gastrointestinal hypersecretion
- **Side effects:**
  - o Anemia
  - o Changes in taste
  - o Confusion
  - o Decreased sperm count
  - o Diarrhea
  - o Dizziness
  - o Headache
  - o Neutropenia
  - o Thrombocytopenia
- **Nursing Intervention:**
  - o Assess the client for confusion (especially elderly clients)
  - o Dilute IV to 2 mL with NaCl and administer over a 2 minute duration
  - o Instruct client to avoid alcohol

- o Instruct client to avoid medications that contain NSAIDs or aspiring
- o Monitor emesis
- o Monitor for blood in stool

Infliximab (Remicade) – anti-rheumatic gastrointestinal anti-inflammatory

- **Action:**
  - o Decrease inflammation in the colon and the joints
- **Side effects:**
  - o Abdominal pain
  - o Acne
  - o Dysuria
  - o Fatigue
  - o Fever
  - o Headache
  - o Infusion reaction
  - o Nausea
  - o Rash
  - o Spot baldness (alopecia)
  - o Upper respiratory infection
  - o Vomiting
- **Nursing intervention:**
  - o Monitor the client for infusion reaction – remember that it can take 2 hours for reaction to show

Magnesium hydroxide/aluminum hydroxide (Maalox, Mylanta, Gaviscon) – antacids

- **Action:**

- o Decreases gas bubbles
- o Neutralizes gastric acid
- **Side effects:**
  - o Constipation
  - o Diarrhea
  - o Increased serum magnesium levels (caused by magnesium hydroxide)
  - o Decreased serum phosphorus levels (caused by aluminum hydroxide)
- **Nursing intervention:**
  - o Destroying the coating of medications that are enteric-coated alters the absorption of these medications (enteric coated means that the drug cannot be dissolved in an acidic environment – it therefore simply passes through the stomach and is dissolved in the intestinal tract which is alkaline)

Mesalamine (Asacol), Olsalaznie (Dipentum) – gastrointestinal anti-inflammatory

- **Action:**
  - o Decrease inflammation of the colon
- **Side effects:**
  - o Dizziness
  - o Headache
  - o Intestinal gas
  - o Malaise
  - o Nausea
  - o Vomiting
  - o Weakness
  - o Mesalamine can cause hair loss, runny nose, pancreatitis, and pharyngitis

- o Olsalazine can cause drug-induced hepatitis and dyscrasias.
- **Nursing intervention:**
  - o Instruct the client to drink 6-8 glasses of fluids every day
  - o Monitor for allergic reactions to sulfa drugs

Metoclopramide (Reglan) – antiemetic

- **Action:**
  - o Increases the rate of gastric emptying
- **Side effects:**
  - o Arrhythmias
  - o Constipation
  - o Diarrhea
  - o Drowsiness
  - o Extrapyramidal reactions
  - o Hypertension or hypotension
  - o Restlessness
- **Nursing intervention:**
  - o Assess the client for tardive dyskinesia
  - o IV should be administered slowly over a 2-minute duration
  - o Monitor the client for extrapyramidal reactions

Midazolam (Versed) – sedative, hypnotic

- **Action:**
  - o Produces depression of the central nervous system
- **Side effects:**
  - o Agitation

- o Drowsiness
- o Apnea
- o Laryngospasm
- o Respiratory depression
- o Hiccups
- o Arrhythmias
- **Nursing intervention:**
    - o Keep resuscitation equipment nearby
    - o Keep reversal medication (Flumazenil (Romazicon)) nearby
    - o Monitor the client for side effects

Misoprostol (Cytotec) – prostaglandin

- **Action:**
    - o Increases protective mucus
    - o Used for antisecretion of gastric acid
- **Side effects:**
    - o Headache
    - o Abdominal pain
    - o Dyspepsia
    - o Intestinal gas
    - o Menstrual disorders
- **Nursing Intervention:**
    - o Monitor emesis
    - o Monitor for blood in stool
    - o Causes spontaneous abortion

Pantoprazole (Protonix) – proton pump inhibitor

- **Action:**
    - o Decreases gastric acid

- **Side effects:**
  - Abdominal pain
  - Diarrhea
  - Headache
  - Increased blood sugar
  - Intestinal gas
- **Nursing Intervention:**
  - Administer the IV dose through a filter over a 15-minute period
  - Assess the client for hememesis
  - Assess the client for melena

<u>**Propofol (Diprivan)**</u> – general anesthetic

- **Action:**
  - Short-acting hypnotic
- **Side effects:**
  - Apnea
  - Bradycardia
  - Dizziness
  - Headache
  - Hypotension
  - Respiratory depression
- **Nursing intervention:**
  - Monitor the client's respirations frequently
  - Prevent contamination from microorganisms (apply aseptic technique when handling the medication)

Above are the most commonly used agents. It is important to note however that other agents can also be used in the treatment of GI disorders. In general, the types of medications used to treat gastrointestinal disorders include the following:

- Antacids
- Antispasmodics
- Antivirals
- Cathartics
- Corticosteroids
- Cytoprotective
- Fiber laxatives
- Hepatitis vaccines
- Histamine receptor blockers
- Immunosuppressives
- Interferons
- Nonsteroidal anti-inflammatory drugs
- Proton pump inhibitors

I hope that you have found this recap helpful. I would recommend reviewing this sections a couple of times until you feel confident that you have remembered most facts. Once you're ready, start testing yourself on realistic practice questions which you can find in the next section. Go over the questions you got wrong, working out why, and start building the winning mindset!

Section 3: Gastrointestinal Practice Questions and Rationales

1. A client with hepatitis C who has just undergone liver biopsy has been admitted to the unit. Which of the following nursing interventions should be performed first?

a. Assess the pre-procedure coagulation studies

b. Perform a chest and abdominal assessment

c. Provide pressure at the site by positioning the client on the right side

d. Provide the patient with discharge instructions

Answer C is correct. After a liver biopsy, the nurse should focus on circulation by applying pressure to the site due to the danger of bleeding. Answer A is incorrect because this is a pre-op priority. Answer B and D are incorrect because these should not be the first action the nurse should take.

2. The nurse receives information on four clients which have been assigned to the hospital. Determine which client needs to be seen first.

a. The client diagnosed with peptic ulcer disease (PUD) who reports epigastric pain

b. The client who was admitted the previous evening and is expelling 275 mL vomitus of c. bright red emesis

d. The client with gastrointestinal bleeding who reports a new episode of melena

e. The post-op client who has undergone cholecystectomy with a temperature of 101.2°F

Answer B is correct. This is because bright red blood in the vomitus indicates an arterial source. The client is at risk of hypovolemia and is therefore a nursing priority. Answer A is incorrect because epigastric pain is a symptom of PUD. Answer C and D are incorrect because although these clients require assessment by the nurse, they are not a priority in this case.

3. The client with severe pancreatitis is being assessed for renal function. Which of the following values would be the best indicator of a complication in this area?

a. Alkaline phosphatase 20U/L

b. BUN 28 mg/dl

c. Creatinine 2.3 mg/dl

d. Hemoglobin 14.6 g/dl

Answer C is correct. This is because creatinine is the most conclusive lab value for assessment of the renal function. The client's creatinine levels are elevated (the normal creatinine level is 0.5–1.5mg/dl) which is indicative of a complication. Answers A and D are incorrect because they are not associated to the kidney. Answer B is also incorrect because although abnormality can relate to kidney function, it is not as conclusive as creatinine.

4. The physician is examining a client with possible appendicitis who has been admitted to the emergency unit. The physician presses downward on the right lower quadrant of the abdomen and asks the client to inform them where the pain is located. The nurse knows that the physician is assessing the client for which of the following?

a. Ascites

b. Rebound tenderness

c. Rovsing's sign

d. Turner's sign

Answer B is correct. This is because rebound tenderness is indicative of peritoneal irritation. The client will experience increased pain when the physician releases pressure in a positive result of this assessment technique. Answer A is incorrect because ascites is a condition of excessive peritoneal fluid in the abdominal cavity which is related to liver disorders. Answer C and D are incorrect because these are signs exhibited by other assessment measures.

5. A client with hepatitis C, who has just undergone liver biopsy, is admitted to the unit. The client is complaining of shortness of breath. Which of the following assessments should the nurse make first?

a. Assessment of the client's mental status

b. Auscultation of breath sounds

c. Liver biopsy site assessment

d. Motor strength and movement of extremities

Answer B is correct. The nurse should firstly verify the client's breath before notifying the surgeon. This is because of the possibility that the lungs may have accidentally been punctured during the surgery. Answers A and D are both incorrect because they are not a priority in this scenario. Answer C is incorrect because although a liver biopsy site assessment is also an important assessment to make, it is not related to the client's shortness of breath.

6. The nurse is preparing for a home visit to a client with hepatitis A. Which of the following would the nurse include on the teaching plan to prevent the client's family from contracting the hepatitis A virus (HAV)?

a. Advise the family to avoid contact with the client's blood

b. Highlight the importance of good hand-washing and personal hygiene

c. Instruct the client to wear a mask at all times

d. Instruct the family to place the client in isolation

Answer B is correct. This is because the HAV is transmitted by the fecal-oral route. Because of this, sanitation, hand-washing and good hygiene are necessary precautions to take to prevent transmission of the HAV. Answer A and C are incorrect because they are not directly associated to hepatitis A. Answer D is incorrect because placing the client in isolation is not necessary.

7. The client with gastrectomy has been admitted to the unit. The nurse expects to administer which of the following vitamins?

a. Ascorbic acid (Ascorba-cap)

b. Cyanocobalamin (Vitamin B12)

c. Phytonadione (Vitamin K)

d. Thiamine (Vitamin B1)

Answer B is correct. This is because the intrinsic factor is reduced following gastrectomy which leads to the poor absorption of vitamin B12. Answers A, C, and D are incorrect because the client's ability to absorb these vitamins is not affected by gastrectomy.

8. The nurse has been assigned to a client with a diagnosis of pancreatitis. Which of the following findings indicates most reliably the presence of of acute pancreatitis?

a. Amylase of 460

b. Hemoglobin of 12.0 g/dL

c. Potassium of 3.1 mEq/L

d. White blood cell count of 14,000

Answer A is correct. This is because assessment of amylase and lipase levels both provide reliable tests which can be used for the diagnosis of pancreatitis. Answer B, C, and D are all incorrect because these findings have no direct correlation to the pancreas.

9. The nurse is assessing a client with long-term cholelithiasis for fat-soluble vitamin deficiencies. Which of the following symptoms would support the diagnosis that the client has a fat-soluble vitamin deficiency?

a. Bleeding gums

b. Constipation

c. Facial numbness

d. Yellow sclera

Answer A is correct. Vitamin A, D, E, and K are the fat-soluble vitamins. Bleeding and bruising are common symptoms that indicate a deficiency in vitamin K. Answers B and C are incorrect because they are not associated with gallstones. Answer D is also incorrect because yellow sclera is a symptom that occurs with the blockage and backup of bile.

10. An elderly client with diverticulitis has been showing symptoms of fever and has been vomiting 12 hours. Which of the following is the best location to measure the client's skin turgor?

a. Back of the arm

b. Dorsal hand

c. Feet

d. Sternum

Answer D is correct. Because of the loss of skin elasticity that occurs with aging, the sternum is the best area to assess elderly clients for skin turgor. Answers A, B, and C are incorrect because these areas are all more affected by the loss of elasticity than the sternum.

11. The client pancreatitis experiencing the process of lipolysis of the pancreas has been admitted to the unit. Given the pathophysiology of lipolysis, which of the following assessments should the nurse prioritize?

a. Assessing breath sounds

b. Assessing for tetany-like movements

c. Examining pedal pulses

d. Obtaining vital signs

Answer B is correct. This is because tetany is indicative of low calcium levels and hypocalcemia is a condition which commonly occurs in clients with pancreatitis and lipolysis. Answer A, C, and D are all relevant assessments but they are not a priority in this case and are therefore incorrect.

12. A pre-op client scheduled for a Nissen repair for a hiatal hernia is being taught to use the incentive spirometer. Which of the following indicates to the nurse that the client has understood the instructions given?

a. "I should do these breathing techniques while lying down flat in bed."

b. "I should use this device once daily."

c. "These exercises will help to decrease my pain."

d. "Using this device will help me to prevent pneumonia."

Answer D is correct. This is because the purpose of incentive spirometer is to treat and prevent atelectasis which can result in pneumonia. Answer A is incorrect because the breathing exercises are best done in the upright sitting position. Answer B is incorrect because patients are generally asked to do many repetitions a day. Answer C is also incorrect because it is a false statement.

13. The nurse caring for a three-day post-op abdominal surgery client. The report the nurse received notes four saturated dressing changes in eight hours. On assessment, dehiscence and evisceration of the client's wound are noted. Which of the following actions should the nurse take after applying a sterile and using a moistened 4x4 gauze?

a. Notify the doctor

b. Place the client in the dorsal recumbent position

c. Transport the client to the treatment room

d. Wrap an Ace bandage around the abdomen

Answer A is correct. The doctor should be notified after applying the saline dressing. Answer B is incorrect because the low Fowler's position should be used, and not the dorsal recumbent position. Answer C is incorrect because transporting the client is an inappropriate action at that time. Answer D is also incorrect because it will not help.

14. The nurse has been assigned to a client with a diagnosis of possible pancreatitis. Which of the following findings best supports a diagnosis of pancreatitis?

a. A serum amylase level of 366 U/L

b. Assessed diminished bowel sounds

c. Client reports passage of fatty stools

d. Pain is in the upper left quadrant of the abdomen

Answer A is correct. This is because assessment of the client's amylase levels is the most indicative when it comes to diagnosis pancreatitis. The client's amylase level in this instance is elevated. Answers B, C, and D are incorrect choices. Although these are also signs of pancreatitis, they are significantly less specific in the diagnosis of pancreatitis.

15. The nursing is preparing the discharge teaching plan to include a high-fiber diet for a client with

diverticulitis. Which of the following dishes would indicate that the client has understood the teaching?

a. Baked chicken and macaroni with cheese

b. Broccoli chicken stir fry with brown rice

c. Broiled liver and dinner roll

d. Spaghetti with meatballs

Answer C is correct. This dish contains the highest amount of fiber and therefore indicates that the client has understood the discharge instructions. Answer A, C, and D are all incorrect because these menu options include very low amounts of fiber and are therefore not recommended.

16. The nurse is assessing a client with a suspected duodenal ulcer. Which of the following diagnostic exams supports a diagnosis of duodenal ulcer?

a. Endoscopic biopsy which indicates a positive H. Pylori

b. Gastric irritation indicated on upper GI

c. Lab results which reveal an elevated WBC count

d. Stool specimen result revealing a positive hemocult

Answer A is correct. Of the above diagnostic exams, the endoscopic biopsy exam is most indicative and most specific to the diagnosis of an ulcer. Answers B, C, and D are incorrect because although these can occur with an ulcer, these exams are not as specific and accurate.

17. The client with a sudden onset of abdominal pain is admitted to the emergency unit. Nursing assessments reveal a bluish discoloration around the umbilicus. Which of the following actions should the nurse take first?

a. Assess the distal pulses

b. Elevate the head of the bed

c. Notify the physician

d. Perform a complete head-to-toe assessment

Answer C is correct. The assessment above describes Cullen's sign and can be indicative of intra-abdominal bleeding. The nurse should immediately notify the physician. Answers A and D are incorrect because they are inappropriate given the scenario. Answer B is also incorrect because changing the position will not rectify the situation.

18. The nurse is preparing a client with gastroesophageal reflux disease (GERD) for discharge. Which food choice would indicate that the client has understood the teaching?

a. Bananas

b. Lemons

c. Oranges

d. Tomatoes

Answer A is correct. This is because clients with GERD should avoid caffeinated beverages, citrus fruits, chocolate, fatty foods, tomato products, and peppermint. Answers B, C, and D are all incorrect because they can lower the LES pressure.

19. A client with a suspected duodenal ulcer being assessed for *H. pylori*. When assessing the client's medical history, the nurse notices a medication which may produce a false negative result. Which one is it?

a. Ampicillin

b. Digoxin (Lanoxin)

c. Ibuprofen (Advil)

d. Propoxyphene napsylate (Darvocet)

Answer A is correct. This is because Ampicillin and other medications such as bismuth preparations (e.g. Pepto-Bismol), histamine blockers (e.g. Tagamet), and proton pump inhibitors (e.g. Prilosec) can affect *H. Pylori* test results. Answers B, C, and D are incorrect because these medications do not affect the test results.

20. The nurse caring for a client with peptic ulcer disease (PUD) and GI bleeding is trying to limit the client's blood loss. Which of the following actions will assist in limiting the amount of blood loss?

a. Administer appropriate medications, such as antacids and histamine blockers

b. Administer blood products as appropriate

c. Monitor the client for fluid loss

d. Monitor the client's vital signs

Answer A is correct. This is because administration of these medications will help with the healing of the ulster as well as assist in avoiding extremes in gastric pH. Answers B, C, and D are all incorrect because these are related to the treatment of hypovolemia.

21. A client with acute diverticulitis is admitted to the unit. Which of the following prescriptions should the nurse question?

a. Cefazolin (Ancef) 1 gm Intravenous piggyback (IVPB) every 8 hours

b. Initiate preparation for a colonoscopy

c. Meperidine (Demerol) 100 mg IM every 4 hours as is required to relieve pain

d. Start IV of normal saline at 100 mL per hour

Answer B is correct. This is because colonoscopies are contraindicated in clients with acute diverticulitis. Answers A, C, and D are incorrect in this case as these are appropriate orders and therefore need not be questioned.

22. The nurse has been assigned to a client who has been admitted to the unit after an MVA. Which of the following findings would indicate to the nurse a possible spleen rupture?

a. Ballance's sign

b. BP 120/70, pulse rate 100, respiration 18

c. Diminished bowel sounds

d. Wheezing on chest auscultation

Answer A is correct. Balance's sign is a dull percussion resonance sound which is heard on the right flank when the client is lying on the left side. It is an indication of ruptured spleen. Answer B is incorrect because it shows normal vital signs. A client with a ruptured spleen would have an elevated heart rate and would exhibit a decreased BP. Answer C is incorrect because although it is related to blood in the abdomen, diminished bowel sounds are not specific to spleen rupture. Answer D is also incorrect because it is not related to spleen rupture.

23. A client with a hiatal hernia has been admitted into the nurse's care after a laparoscopic Nissen fundoplication (LNF). Which of the following should the client avoid if gas-bloat syndrome occurs?

a. Antireflux medications

b. Beef or red meats

c. Carbonated beverages

d. Exercise

Answer C is correct. When clients are unable to or have difficulties belching, this may lead to gas-bloat syndrome. Clients should therefore avoid carbonated beverages as well as any gas-causing foods such as beans, broccoli, and cabbage. Answers A, B, and D are incorrect because these do not contribute to the gas formation.

24. The nurse is assigning tasks for a client who has been admitted with acute pancreatitis. Which would of the following actions can the nurse assign to the nurse's assistant?

a. Administer medications to relieve pain

b. Monitor NG drainage for amount, character, and color

c. Provide oral hygiene every 2 hours

d. Teach the client to assume the fetal position in order to relieve pain

Answer C is correct. This is personal hygiene and comfort measures may be provided by assistive personnel. Answers A, B, and D are incorrect because these are all actions which can be performed by licensed personnel only.

25. The RN is acting as preceptor to a newly licensed RN. Which of the following actions by the new RN would require preceptor intervention?

a. Assisting a two-day post-op client to ambulate in the hallway

b. Performing an abdominal assessment by auscultating bowel sounds

c. Preparation for manipulation of an NG tube on a client 2 hours post-op bariatric surgery

d. Teaching a client to splint the surgical site during coughing and deep breathing exercises

Answer C is correct. This is because manipulation of the NG tube can disrupt the anastomosis or the suture line on this client. The physician should immediately be notified if there is reason to believe that there has been a disruption of the tube. Answers A, B, and D are all incorrect in this case because they are all correct nursing actions and therefore do not require preceptor intervention.

26. A client with a possible appendicitis is admitted to the unit. Which of the following diagnostic test results will best assist in confirming the diagnosis?

a. A normal CT scan

b. An elevated sedimentation rate

c. Ultrasound revealing an enlarged appendix

d. WBC count of 16,000/mm with a shift to the left

Answer C is correct. Ultrasounds which reveal an enlarged appendix will provide the best diagnostic evaluation. Answer A is incorrect because the CT scan would be abnormal with appendicitis. Answer B and D are also incorrect because even though they could technically occur with appendicitis, they are not as conclusive as the ultrasound.

27. The nurse is helping the doctor with a paracentesis procedure on a client with cirrhosis of the liver. Which of the following actions would the nurse take first?

a. Identify the client

b. Instruct the client to empty the bladder

c. Obtain consent

d. Place the client in a sitting position

Answer A is correct. Identification of the client should be the first step when performing any procedure. Following this, the nurse should obtain consent (C), then instruct the client to empty the bladder (B), and then the nurse should place the client in a sitting position (D).

28. The nurse has been assigned to a client with cholecystitis. Which of the following symptoms would the nurse expect the client to exhibit?

a. Bradycardia

b. Dysphagia

c. Fever

d. Hiccups

Answer C is correct. Other symptoms of cholecystitis include nausea, pain, vomiting, indigestion, intestinal gas, and rebound tenderness upon palpation. Answer A, B, and D are all incorrect because these are note symptoms that are associated with cholecystitis.

29. A client has an esophageal balloon in place for bleeding esophageal varices. Which of the following must be kept at the client's bedside?

a. Emesis basin

b. Mouth swabs

c. Scissors

d. Tracheostomy

Answer C is correct. This is because if the balloon slips upwards, obstructing the client's airway, the scissors are necessary to cut the tube. Answers A and B are incorrect because these are not essential and are rather used for comfort measures. Answer D is also incorrect because a tracheostomy is unnecessary.

30. The nurse is preparing to care for a client following conventional surgery for a sliding hiatal hernia. Which of the following nursing interventions should the nurse prioritize?

a. Assessing the dressing site for bleeding

b. Monitoring for abdominal pain and medicating appropriately

c. Monitoring the NG tube for patency and repositioning the tube if it is not working properly

d. Teaching the client how to use the incentive spirometry and making sure that it is used appropriately

Answer D is correct. Because of the risk of respiratory complications, any interventions relating to the respiratory system should be made a priority. Answers A and B are incorrect because although appropriate, they are not the priority in this scenario. Answer C is incorrect because of the repositioning the tube should not be attempted due to the danger of perforation.

31. A client who has completed a gastroscopy procedure has been diagnosed with GERD. Which instructions should the nurse include on the client's teaching plan?

a. Avoid alcohol and tobacco

b. Eat a snack everyday at bedtime

c. Eat regular meals three times a day

d. Resume the recumbent position after meals

Answer A is correct. The client should be instructed to avoid anything which lowers the LES, including tobacco and alcohol. Answers B is incorrect because food should be avoided 2-3 hours before bedtime. Answer C is incorrect because the client should be instructed to consume 4 to 6 small meals per day. Answer D is also incorrect because the client should be taught to remain upright for 1-2 hours after meals.

32. A client with an ulcer has undergone Billroth II procedure two days ago. Which of the following actions should the nurse take in order to prevent dumping syndrome?

a. Serve high-volume meal contents

b. Provide a diet which is low-carbohydrate, high-protein, and high-fat

c. Encourage the client to drink at least 500 mL of fluids with meals

d. Elevate the client's head of the bed 45° after meals

Answer B is correct. This is because rapid emptying of gastric contents into the small intestine is thought to be one of the causes of dumping syndrome. Therefore, a diet which is low-carbohydrate, high-protein, and high-fat will serve to decrease the incidence of dumping syndrome. Answer A is incorrect because the client should be ingesting small amounts at each meal. Answer C is incorrect because the client cannot consume liquids when eating. Answer D is also incorrect because the client should lie down after meals.

33. A client with a nasogastric tube in place has been assigned to the nurse's care. Assessment of the aspirate reveals a pH of 2.0. Which of the following is the appropriate nursing intervention?

a. Turn the client side lying and reassess the aspirate

b. Remove the NG tube and replace it

c. Notify the physician

d. Document the finding

Answer D is correct. This is because the finding is within the normal range. The normal value for gastric aspirate is 0-4. Answers A, B, and C are incorrect because these are not necessary due to the fact that it is a normal reading.

34. A client with an ulcer has been placed on tetracycline after a positive helicobacter pyloric test result. Which of the following, if taken with the medication, would decrease the effectiveness of the medication?

a. Bananas

b. Bran cereal

c. Cabbage

d. Yogurt

Answer D is correct. This is because, when taken at the same time, milk and dairy products can reduce the effectiveness of tetracycline. Answers A, B, and C are incorrect because they do not affect the effectiveness of the medication.

35. A client with hepatitis C has been scheduled for a liver biopsy. Which of the following findings in the client's record should receive priority?

a. BUN of 22 mg/dl

b. Hematocrit 42%

c. Potassium 4.0 mEq/L

d. Prothrombin time of 56 seconds

Answer D is correct. This is because an abnormal prothrombin time would incur the risk of hemorrhage with a liver biopsy. It should therefore receive priority.

Answers A, B, and C are incorrect because these are all normal values and therefore do not incur any procure risks.

36. The client with pancreatitis who has been admitted to the medical surgical unit is complaining of dyspnea. Which of the following is the appropriate initial nursing action?

a. Assess the client for vital signs and record them in the client's medical record

b. Elevate the head of the bed

c. Instruct the client to breathe in through the mouth and out via the nostrils

d. Notify the healthcare provider

Answer B is correct. This is because elevating the client's head of the bed will relieve pressure from the abdomen, thereby facilitating the client's breathing ability.
Answers A and C are incorrect because they are not effective in relieving dyspnea. Answer D is also incorrect because notifying the healthcare provider should not be the initial action.

37. A client with a diagnosis of end-stage liver disease is admitted to the unit. Which of the following tasks can the nurse delegate to the UAP?

a. Administer the antacid

b. Assess the client's skin for signs of breakdown

c. Evaluate the degree of ascites

d. Obtain dressing supplies for the room from a provided list

Answer D is correct. A UAP can obtain dressing supplies from a provided list. Answers A, B, and D are incorrect because these actions require nursing skills which cannot be taken by the UAP.

38. A client with cirrhosis of the liver returns to the unit after a banding procedure for esophageal varices. Which of the following complaints should the nurse report to the physician?

a. Chest pain

b. Drowsiness

c. Eructation

d. Nausea

Answer A is correct. The nurse should be concerned if the client complaints of chest pain and immediately notify the physician. This is because the banding procedure could cause ulceration of the mucosa and bleeding. Answers B and C are incorrect because these are expected side effects associated to the procedure. Answer D is incorrect because even though the nurse should assess the client should the client be feeling nauseous, it is not a priority in this case.

39. The nurse is preparing a client diagnosed with GERD for discharge. Which of the following statements by the client indicates to the nurse a need for further teaching?

a. "Because I am overweight, I need to follow a weight reduction diet."

b. "I need to remain upright for one to two hours after meals."

c. "I should avoid wearing tight-fitting clothes."

d. "I should eat three large meals per day."

Answer D is correct. This is because clients with GERD are instructed to have 4 to 6 small meals every day in order to prevent reflux. Answers A, B, and C are incorrect because these are correct recommendations which are given to clients to control reflux. Other instructions the nurse should include on the teaching plan include: avoidance of food 2-3 hours before bedtime, avoidance of snacks in the evening, elevation of the head at nighttime, avoidance of straining and heavy lifting, and elimination of alcohol, coffee, carbonated drinks, chocolate, fatty and spiced foods.

40. A client has been admitted to the unit after an open surgical procedure for a hiatal hernia repair. Which of the following interventions should the nurse prioritize?

a. Administering pain medication as required

b. Assisting with and monitoring incentive spirometry

c. Lowering the head of the bed to prevent hypovolemia

d. Monitoring the client for bladder distention every four hours

Answer B is correct. This is because after an open procedure to repair a hiatal hernia, nursing intervention should focus on preventing any respiratory complications. The nurse should therefore teach the client how to use the incentive spirometer and monitor its correct use because the incentive spirometer encourages deep breathing and lung expansion.

41. The client with a suspected diagnosis of peptic ulcer disease (PUD) reports epigastric pain after eating. The physician orders a urea breath test for *H. pylori*. Which of the following should the nurse include in the client's teaching plan for test preparation?

a. Asking the client to bring a sputum sample with her for analysis

b. Clear liquids the day before the test

c. High-fat meal two hours before the test

d. Withhold oral food and fluids the night before the test

Answer D is correct. NPO is the only preparation for a *H. pylori* urea breath test. The client should therefore be instructed not to eat and not to drink the night before his test. During the urea breath test for *H. pylori*, the client will be asked to drink a carbon-enriched urea liquid and the CO_2 is then measured for *H. pylori*. Answers A, B, and C are all incorrect because these are not preparations which have to be taken for the *H. pylori* urea breath test.

42. A client has been admitted into the nurse's care after a gastroscopy procedure where he received midazolam HCl (Versed) and propofol (Diprivan). Following assessment, the nurse notes a heart rate of 110 and an O₂ saturation of 75, BP 88/40. Which of the following should the nurse prioritize?

a. Decrease the heart rate

b. Increase the blood pressure

c. Increase the O2 saturation levels

d. Prevent aspiration

Answer C is correct. This is because from the values given, the client is experiencing severe O2 deficiency and therefore the first action to be taken by the nurse is t increase the O2 saturation levels (the normal O2 saturation value is 95-100). Answer A is incorrect because it is not an immediate priority in this case. Oxygenation should be the nurse's primary focus given the scenario. Answer B is incorrect because increasing blood pressure is again not a priority. Answer D is incorrect because there is no evidence that the client is at an increased risk of aspiration.

43. The physician has ordered lactulose (Cephalac) for a client with cirrhosis of the liver. Which of the following indicates to the nurse that the medication is having its intended effect?

a. A generalized increase in bruising

b. An increase in bowel movements

c. Hypoactive bowel sounds

d. The client sleeping more

Answer B is correct. This is because the effect of lactulose is to promote the movement of ammonia from the blood into the colon. An increase in bowel movement is therefore an indication that the medication is have its indented effect of eliminating ammonia. Answer A and C are incorrect because these are not associated to lactulose. Answer D is also incorrect because this would indicate a build-up of ammonia in the blood which means the client's situation is worsening, not improving.

44. The client with pancreatitis on the previous shift is admitted to the unit. Upon evaluating the laboratory results, which of the following values would indicate to the nurse that immediate intervention is required?

a. Potassium 4.0 mEq/L

b. Serum amylase 300 units/dL

c. Sodium 120 mEq/L

d. White blood cell 12,000 cells/mm

Answer C is correct. This is because the sodium value given is extremely low (normal sodium level ranges between 135–145 mEq/L). Immediate intervention is therefore necessary. Answer A is incorrect because the value given is within the normal range which is 3.5–5.0 mEq/L for potassium. Answer B is also incorrect because although the serum amylase is above the normal level, which is 60–160 units/L, an elevated serum amylase is an expected side effect of pancreatitis and immediate intervention is therefore not necessary. answer D is also incorrect because although there is a slight elevation in the client's white blood cells, the normal range being between 5,000 and 10,000 cells/mm, it is not a priority in this case.

45. The nurse has been assigned to a three-day post-op client with acute diverticulitis who has undergone a bowel resection and colostomy. Which of the following post-op assessment findings should the nurse immediately report to the physician?

a. Absence of feces in the colostomy bag

b. Gray dusky color of the stoma

c. Mucus oozing from the stoma opening

d. Stoma protrudes above the abdominal wall

Answer B is correct. This is because a gray dusky color is an indication of necrosis which the nurse should immediately report to the doctor. Answer A is incorrect because it can take 2 to 4 days for the colostomy to function. Answers C and D are both also incorrect because these are normal findings.

46. The nurse is caring for a client with cirrhosis and bleeding esophageal varices who has a Sengstaken-Blakemore tube in place. Which of the following assessment assessment findings should the nurse prioritize?

a. Blood noted in the lumen that is in the stomach

b. Blood pressure elevation by 20 mm/Hg

c. The label is missing from one of the three tube lumens

d. Wheezing on chest auscultation

Answer D is correct. This is because when using the Sengstaken-Blakemore tube, aspiration and airway occlusion are the most dangerous complications that can occur and therefore require immediate intervention. Answer A is incorrect because this is an expected side effect. Answer B and C are also incorrect because although they require further nursing intervention, they are not a priority in this case.

47. A client arrives at the clinic complaining of difficult swallowing and heartburn. A tentative diagnosis of GERD. Which of the following symptoms would further support this diagnosis?

a. Blood in the stool

b. Dryness of the mouth

c. Globus

d. Vomiting

Answer C is correct. This is because Globus, i.e. a feeling that something is in the back of the throat, is a common symptom in clients with GERD. Answers A, B, and D are incorrect because these are not symptoms which are associated with GERD.

48. The nurse has been assigned to a client with cholecystitis. The nurse expects the client to be exhibiting which of the following symptoms?

a. Bradycardia

b. Dysphagia

c. Fever

d. Hiccups

Answer C is correct. This is because fever, flatulence, nausea, pain, vomiting, indigestion, and tenderness upon palpation are all symptoms associated with cholecystitis. Answers A, B, and D are incorrect because these are not symptoms associated with cholecystitis.

49. The client with cirrhosis of the liver and fluid in the peritoneal cavity is admitted to the hospital. The doctor instructs the nurse to prepare the client for a paracentesis. Which of the following interventions should the nurse include in the preparation plan?

a. Assessing that the client empties the bladder

b. Obtaining a lipid profile

c. Placing the client in the prone position

d. Starting an IV with an 18-gauge needle

Answer A is correct. This is because for a paracentesis procedure, the bladder should be emptied in order to prevent incidental puncturing. Answer B and D are incorrect because these are note necessary interventions. Answer C is also incorrect because during the procedure, the client should be sat upright, and not in the prone position.

50. The nurse is preparing a client with diverticulosis who has been ordered a high-fiber diet for discharge. Which of the following dish selections would indicate to the nurse that the client has understood the teaching?

a. Beef broth

b. Froot Loops cereal with milk

c. Sliced turkey on white bread

d. Spinach salad

Answer D is correct. This is because spinach contains a lot of fiber and is therefore a good choice. Answers A, B, and C are all incorrect because these dishes contain very little fiber.

51. The nurse is preparing a client with a percutaneous gastrostomy tube for discharge. Which of the following indicates that the client's family has understood the teaching plan?

a. "If my mother is unable to swallow, I will discontinue the feeding and call the clinic immediately."

b. "I will report any signs of indigestion to the physician."

c. "I must check placement four times every day."

d. "After meals, I must flush the tube with water and clamp the tube."

Answer D is correct. This is because the client's family should be instructed to flush the tube with water and camp the tube after meals. Answer A is incorrect because no swallowing is required as the tube is inserted in the stomach. Answer B is incorrect because indigestion is something that can occur with the percutaneous gastronomy tube. The client can receive a prescription for indigestion but this is by no means a reason for alarm. Answer C is also incorrect because the placement should be check prior to feedings.

52. The client who has been placed on Amphotericin B has been admitted to the unit. Which of the following symptoms indicates to the nurse that the client is experiencing toxicity to the medication?

a. Changes in skin color

b. Changes in vision

c. Nausea

d. Urinary frequency

Answer A is correct. Because Amphotericin B is toxic to the kidneys and liver and can cause bone marrow suppression, clients who are receiving this medication should be monitored frequently for bone marrow, liver, and renal function. Yellowing skin or jaundice, although not specific to the use of the medication, is a symptom of liver toxicity. Answers B, C, and D are all incorrect because changes in vision, nausea, and urinary frequency are not signs of toxicity.

53. The physician has ordered Exelon (rivastigmine) for the client with Alzheimer's disease. Which of the following side effects can the nurse expect the client to exhibit?

a. Confusion
b. GI upset
c. Headaches
d. Urinary incontinence

Answer B is correct. This is because gastrointestinal upset and nausea are symptoms most commonly associated with acetylcholinesterase inhibitors such as Exelon. Other clinical manifestations include clumsiness, dizziness, toxicity, and unsteadiness. Answer A is incorrect because clients with Alzheimer's will already be experiencing confusion. Answer C and D are also incorrect because although the client may be experiencing headaches and urinary incontinence, these symptoms are not necessary associated with the medication.

54. The nurse has been assigned to a client with uremic frost. The nurse knows that uremic frost is often seen in

clients with which of the following conditions?

a. Arteriosclerosis

b. Liver failure

c. Parathyroid disorder

d. Severe anemia

Answer B is correct. This is because uremic frost is most common in clients with liver disease. Answers A, C, and D are all incorrect because uremic frost is not related to arteriosclerosis, parathyroid disorders, or anemia.

55. The nurse is caring for a client with pancreatic cancer who has been admitted to the unit after a Whipple procedure. The nurse understands that during the Whipple procedure, the doctor removes which of the following?

a. The head of the pancreas
b. The jejunum and the esophagus
c. The proximal third section of the small intestines
d. The stomach and the duodenum

Answer A is correct. The head of the pancreas, a portion of the stomach, and the jejunum are removed and reanastomosed during a Whipple procedure. Answer B is incorrect because the esophagus is not removed. Answer C is incorrect because the proximal third of the small intestine is not removed. Answer D is also incorrect because the entire stomach is not removed during the procedure.

56. The client with an abdominal cholecystectomy is admitted to the unit after a surgery with a Jackson-Pratt drain. The Jackson-Pratt drain is utilized for which purpose?

a. To keep the common bile duct open
b. To prevent the need for dressing changes
c. To provide for wound drainage
d. To reduce edema at the incision

Answer C is correct. This is because a Jackson-Pratt drain is a serum-collection device which is utilized during abdominal surgery in order to provide wound drainage. Answer A is incorrect because a t-tube is used to keep the common bile duct open. Answer B and D are also incorrect because the Jackson-Pratt drain will not prevent nor reduce the need for dressing changes, nor will it reduce edema at the incision.

57. The nurse is caring for a client with acute pancreatitis who is experiencing severe abdominal pain. Which of the following prescriptions should the nurse question?

a. Cimetadine 300mg PO m.i.d.

b. Meperidine 100mg IM m 4 hours PRN pain

c. Morphine 8mg IM m 4 hours PRN pain

d. Mylanta 30 ccs m 4 hours via NG

Answer C is correct. This is because morphine causes spasms of the Sphincter of Oddi and is contraindicated in clients with pancreatitis and in clients with gallbladder disease. The nurse should therefore question this order. Answers A, B, and D are all incorrect because

Cimetadine Meperidine, and Mylanta are all medications which are ordered for clients with pancreatitis.

58. The nurse is caring for a client with renal failure. Given his conditions, the client is to be placed on a low potassium diet. Which of the following would be the best meal choice for the client?

a. 1 cup beef broth

b. 1 cup rice

c. ½ cup raisins

d. 2 baked potatoes with the skin

Answer B is correct. This is because rice is low in potassium and is therefore a good food choice for the client with renal failure. Answers A, C, and D are all incorrect because these all contain high amounts of potassium which the client should avoid.

59. The male client who has just undergone a recent liver transplant inquires for how long he would need to be taking immunosuppressant. What answer should the nurse give?

a. For one year

b. For the next decade

c. For the next seven years

d. For the rest of his life

Answer D is correct. This is because clients with liver transplants will have to be maintained on immunosuppressants for the rest of their lives. Answers A, B, and C are therefore all incorrect.

60. The physician has ordered Lactulose for a client with cirrhosis of the liver. The nurse knows that Lactulose is prescribed in order to:

a. Lower the client's ammonia level

b. Lower the client's blood glucose level

c. Lower the client's uric acid level

d. Lower the creatinine level in the serum

Answer A is correct. The is because the medication is administered in order to lower the ammonia levels in clients with cirrhosis. Answers B, C, and D are therefore incorrect because the intended effect of Lactulose is not to lower blood glucose levels, nor the uric acid levels, nor the client's creatinine levels.

61. The client with cancer of the liver has been admitted to the oncology unit. Which of the following findings should the nurse be most concerned about?

a. An alteration in nutrition

b. An alteration in urinary elimination

c. An alteration in skin integrity

d. Ineffective coping

Answer A is correct. This is because liver cancer often results in severe vomiting and nausea and therefore the requirement to alter nutrition. Answers B, C, and D are incorrect because they are not a nursing priority in this case.

62. The nurse is working with a patient care assistant and another nurse. Which of the following clients should the nurse assign to the registered nurse?

a. The client who received post-thyroidectomy a week ago

b. The three-day post-splenectomy client

c. The two-day post-appendectomy client

d. The two-day post-thoracotomy client

Answer D is correct. The post-thoracotomy client should be assigned to the registered nurse because this is the most crucial client. Answers A and C are incorrect because these clients are ready to be discharged. Answer B is also incorrect because this client is stable enough three days after the splenectomy and can therefore be assigned to the PN nurse.

63. The adolescent client with appendicitis has been admitted to the hospital. The client's parents, who are Jehovah's Witnesses, refuse to sign the blood permit. Which of the following nursing actions is most appropriate?

a. Notify the doctor of the refusal

b. Explain the consequences without treatment

c. Encourage them to change their mind

d. Administer the blood without permission

Answer A is correct. The nurse should notify the doctor if the client's parents refuse to sign the blood permit. The court might order treatment because the client is still a minor. Answers B and C are incorrect because it is not the responsibility of the nurse to persuade or explain the potential consequences to the client's parents. Answer D is also incorrect because the legal guardians of the client have the right to refuse the blood transfusion.

64. The nurse is caring for a client who has been admitted to the unit after a cholescystectomy. The nurse knows that Montgomery straps are used on this client because:

a. The client will require frequent dressing changes

b. The client is at risk for evisceration

c. No sutures or clips are used to secure the incision

d. Montgomery straps provide support for drains that are inserted into the incision

Answer A is correct. This is because clients who have received a cholecystectomy will often have a lot of draining on the dressing. Montgomery straps are therefore used in order to secure dressings that require frequent dressing changes. Answer B is incorrect because the client is not at a higher higher risk of evisceration. Answer C is incorrect because clips or sutures are used to secure the wounds of clients who have undergone cholescystectomy. Answer D is also incorrect because these straps are not used to support drains that are inserted into the incision.

65. The nurse is preparing a client with cirrhosis for pericentesis. Which of the following instructions should the nurse give to the client before the exam?

"You will need to lay down flat during the procedure."

"You will be asleep during the whole procedure."

"You need to empty your bladder before the exam."

"During the exam, the doctor will inject a medication to treat your illness."

Answer C is correct. The nurse should instruct the client to empty the bladder before the pericentesis in order to prevent the risk of puncturing of the bladder. Answer A is incorrect because the client will be leaning over an over the bed table or in a sitting up position. Answer B is incorrect because clients are awake during the exam. Answer D is also incorrect because medications are not usually administered during the procedure.

66. The client with a diagnosis of hepatitis who is experiencing pruritus has been assigned into the nurse's care. Which of the following is the most appropriate nursing intervention?

a. Encourage the client take warm showers twice daily

b. Encourage a hot-water rinse after bathing

c. Apply powder to the client's skin

d. Add baby oil to the client's bath water

Answer D is correct. Pruritus is severe itching of the skin. Because of this, it is recommended to add baby oils to the client's bath water to sooth the skin. Oils can also be applied to dry skin in order to help alleviate the itching. Answer A is incorrect because frequent showering can cause the skin to become even dryer. Answer B is incorrect because rinsing with hot water also dries out the skin. Answer D is also incorrect because baby powder too, contributes to dry skin.

67. The nurse is caring for a female client with cancer of the pancreas and is taking her vital signs. Which of the following is the fifth vital sign?

a. Anorexia

b. Fatigue

c. Insomnia

d. Pain

Answer D is correct. Pain is the fifth vital sign. When taking the client's vital sigs, the nurse should assess and record the client's blood pressure, pain levels, pulse, and temperature. Answers A, B, and C are incorrect. Although these are included in the charting, they are not considered to be the fifth vital sign.

68. The nurse has been assigned to a client with pancreatitis who has been admitted to the intensive care unit. Which of the following orders should the nurse anticipate?

a. Change dressing twice daily

b. Insert a Levine tube

c. Monitor the client's cardiac activity

d. Take the client's blood pressure every 15 minutes

Answer B is correct. Clients with pancreatitis often experience vomiting and nausea. The nurse should therefore expect to insert a Levine tube because lavage is frequently used to decompress the stomach and rest the bowel. Answer A is incorrect because changing the client's dressing is not required. Answers C is incorrect because although cardiac monitoring may be needed, this order is not specific to the client with pancreatitis. Answer D is also incorrect because the client's blood pressure doesn't need to be measured every 15 minutes.

69. The nurse is preparing a client with diverticulitis who has been placed on a low-roughage diet for discharge. The client should be instructed to avoid which of the following?

a. Chicken

b. Cooked broccoli

c. Custard

d. Noodles

Answer B is correct. This is because clients with diverticulitis should be instructed to avoid eating gas-causing foods like cooked broccoli which will only serve to exacerbate abdominal discomfort. Answers A, C, and D are incorrect because these foods can be included on the client's diet.

70. The nurse is caring for a client who has just undergone hemorrhoidectomy. Which of the following diets is most appropriate?

a. Bland

b. Clear-liquid

c. High-fiber

d. Lactose free

Answer B is correct. A client who has just undergone surgery should receive a clear-liquid diet. The client should slowly be introduced into a regular diet. In order to avoid constipation, stool softeners may also be administered as part of the client's care plan. Answer C is incorrect for because a client who has just undergone hemorrhoidectomy should not be placed on a high-fiber diet straight away. A high-fiber diet should however be encouraged later on. Answer A and D are incorrect because these are not diets that are included in the postoperative care after hemorrhoidectomy.

71. Which of the following should to nurse reinforce when teaching about irritable bowel syndrome (IBS)?

a. The need to instruct clients to limit the intake of fruits and vegetables

b. The need to instruct clients to adopt a low-fiber diet

c. The need to encourage clients to drink 16 ounces of fluid with each meal

d. The need for a balanced high-nutrient and high-fiber diet

Answer D is correct. When teaching about IBS, the nurse should reinforce the need for a balanced diet which is at the same time high in nutrients and high in fiber. Clients with IBS should avoid foods which cause or contribute to bloating and diarrhea, such as alcohol, caffeinated beverages, fried food and spicy food. Answers A and B are incorrect because these are wrong teachings. Answer C is also incorrect because it is not necessary.

72. The nurse has been assigned to a client who complaints of stomach ache which arises roughly two hours after meals. Which of the following conditions should the nurse expect?

a. Peptic ulcer
b. Gastric ulcer
c. Duodenal ulcer
d. Curling's ulcer

Answer C is correct. This is because pain which arises 2-3 hours after meals is associated to clients with duodenal ulcers. In these clients, eating often helps to relieve pain. Answer A is incorrect because it is too vague and fails to distinguish the ulcer. Answer B is incorrect because clients with gastric ulcers will usually experience pain approximately 30 minutes after eating. Answer D is also incorrect because Curling's ulcer is an ulcer that is associated with stress, also called Curling's stress ulcer.

73. The nurse has been assigned to a patient with ulcerative colitis. Which of the following nursing diagnoses should the nurse prioritize?

a. Altered nutritional requirements

b. Anxiety

c. Fluid volume deficit

d. Impaired skin integrity

Answer C is correct. The nurse should prioritize the fluid volume deficit because fluid volume deficit can lead to electrolyte loss and metabolic acidosis. Answer A, B, and D are incorrect because although they may be applicable in this case, these are not a priority.

74. The physician has ordered metronidazole (Flagyl) for adjunct treatment for a patient with duodenal ulcer. Which of the following should the nurse include on the teaching plan?

a. "Avoid alcohol while taking this medication."

b. "Take the medication on an empty stomach in order to facilitate absorption."

c. "Take the medication only until you start feeling better."

d. "While taking the medication, you do not need to be concerned about being exposed to the sun."

Answer A is correct. The client should be instructed to avoid alcoholic beverages when taking the medication because alcohol, when consumed with Flagyl, can result in extreme nausea. Answer B is incorrect because the medication should be taken with a full glass of water during meals. Answer C is also incorrect because the client should be instructed to complete the course of treatment. Answer D is also incorrect because Flagyl will often cause the client to become photosensitive and the client should therefore be instructed to avoid direct sunlight when taking the medication.

75. The nurse is caring for a client who inquires whether peptic ulcers are caused by stress. Which of the following is the appropriate answer the nurse should provide?

a. "Peptic ulcers are always caused from exposure to regular stress."

b. "Peptic ulcers are associated with the *H. pylori* virus, although there are other ulcers that can be related to stress."

c. "Peptic ulcers are caused by excessive consumption of fatty foods."

d. "Peptic ulcers, like all ulcers, result from stress."

Answer B is correct. This is because peptic ulcers are not always associated with stress, although stress can be a component of the disease. Answers A and C are incorrect because the statements are both untrue. Answer D is also incorrect because peptic ulcers are associated but not directly caused by stress.

76. The client with hepatitis A is admitted to the hospital. When assessing the client's medical history, the nurse notices that one of the client's regular medications is contraindicated due to the HAV. Which

of the following medications is the nurse referring to?

a. Lipitor (atorvastatin)

b. Premarin (conjugated estrogens)

c. Prilosec (omeprazole)

d. Synthroid (levothyroxine)

Answer A is correct. This is because lipid-lowering agents such as Lipitor are contraindicated in clients with active liver diseases. Answers B, C, and D are incorrect because these medications are not contraindicated by the HAV.

77. A client with suspected acute pancreatitis is admitted to the hospital. Which of the following laboratory finding confirms the diagnosis for acute pancreatitis?

a. Blood glucose of 255mg/dL

b. Platelet count of 250,000cu/mm

c. Serum amylase level of 500 units/dL

d. White cell count of 22,000cu/mm

Answer C is correct. This is because laboratory values revealing a serum amylase levels greater than 200 units/dL is indicative of acute pancreatitis and can therefore help in the diagnosis. Answer A is incorrect because elevations of blood glucose levels are not specific to acute pancreatitis. Answer B is incorrect because the platelet count given is within the normal range and therefore doesn't help in the diagnosis. Answer D is incorrect because elevations in white cell count occur in conditions other than acute pancreatitis.

78. The client with diverticulitis is admitted to the hospital with dehydration, nausea, and vomiting. Which of the following findings suggests to the nurse that there may be a complication relating to diverticulitis?

a. Abdominal distention

b. A rigid abdomen

c. Signs of fever

d. Pain in the left lower quadrant

Answer B is correct. This is because a board-like and rigid abdomen can be an indication of peritonitis. Peritonitis is a complication of diverticulitis. Answers A, C, and D are incorrect because these are all common findings in clients with diverticulitis.

79. The nurse is caring for a client with primary sclerosing cholangitis who was admitted to the unit after a liver transplant. When assessing the client for complications, the nurse notices a finding which may be indicative of a post-transplant complication. Which

of the following findings would indicate acute rejection of the new liver?

a. Abdominal distention and stools which are clay in color

b. Elevated creatinine levels and increased uric acid

c. Foul-smelling bile drainage and fever

d. Yellowed skin and prolonged prothrombin time

Answer D is correct. This is because prolonged prothrombin time and jaundice are both signs that the new liver isn't working. The nurse should immediately report these findings to the physician. Answer A is incorrect because abdominal distention and stools which are clay in color are symptoms which are associated with obstruction. Answer B is incorrect because elevated creatinine levels and increased uric acid are symptoms related to renal failure. And answer C is also incorrect because foul-smelling bile and fever are symptoms which are associated with an infection.

80. The nurse has been assigned to a client who has just undergone laparoscopic cholecystectomy. Which of the following discharge instructions should the nurse include on the teaching plan?

a. "Should you experience any pain in the back or shoulders, you should immediately report this to the clinic."

b. "Expect your abdominal pain to decrease over the course of the next week."

c. "Expect to experience stools that are clay-colored."

d. "Avoid taking a bath for the next 48 hours."

Answer D is correct. This is because clients should avoid taking a bath for 48 hours after a laparoscopic cholecystectomy and this should therefore be included in the nurse's teaching plan. Answer A is incorrect because pain in the back and shoulders is an expected side effect. Answer B is incorrect because the pain will not be located in the stomach, but in the shoulders. Answer C is also incorrect because stools should not be clay-colored following the laparoscopic cholecystectomy.

81. The nurse is caring for an 8-year-old client who is has been scheduled for a cholecystectomy. The nurse should question which of the following drug prescriptions?

a. Tagamet (cimetadine)

b. Phenergan (promethazine)

c. Demerol (meperidine)

d. Atropine (atropine)

Answer D is correct. This is because Atropine causes an increase in intraocular pressure and is therefore contraindicated in clients with glaucoma. Because of this, the nurse should question the prescription for Atropine. Answer A, B, and C are all incorrect because these medications are not contraindicated in clients with glaucoma.

82. The nurse is caring for a client with fever, diarrhea, and abdominal pain. Prior to assessing the client, the nurse notices that the client has a history of diverticulitis. Which of the following foods has caused the client's symptoms?

a. Baked fish

b. Mashed potatoes

c. Steamed carrots

d. Whole-grain cereal

Answer D is correct. This is because ingestion of foods such as celery, nuts, popcorn, raw vegetables and whole grans is known to cause symptoms related to diverticulitis. Answers A, B, and C are all incorrect because these types of food are not known to cause the given symptoms in clients with diverticulitis.

83. The client with irritable bowel syndrome has been admitted to the unit. Which of the following is indicative of irritable bowel syndrome?

a. Alternating spells of diarrhea and constipation

b. Development of pouches in the wall of the intestine

c. Hypocalcemia and iron-deficiency anemia

d. Thickening, swelling, and abscess formation

Answer A is correct. This is because clients with irritable bowel syndrome will experience spells of diarrhea and constipation. Answer B is incorrect because the development of pouches in the inner wall of the intestine is a symptom associated with diverticulosis. Answer C is incorrect because because both hypocalcemia and iron-deficiency anemia are symptoms related to ulcerative colitis. Answer D is also incorrect because thickening, swelling, and abscess formation are all symptoms which are associated with Crohn's disease.

84. The nurse has been assigned to a client with acute pancreatitis. When preparing the client's caring plan, which of the following diets should the nurse encourage?

a. High carbohydrate and low protein

b. High fat and high protein

c. Low calorie and low carbohydrate

d. Low fat and high calorie

Answer D is correct. This is because clients with acute pancreatitis should be placed on a diet that is low in fat and high calorie. Answers A, B, and C are all incorrect because these diets will only service to exacerbate the client's discomfort.

85. The doctor has ordered a blood test for *H. pylori*. In preparing the client for the test, the nurse should:

a. Administer an oral suspension of glucose one hour before the test is scheduled

b. Explain to the client that a small dose of radioactive isotope will be used during the exam

c. Inform the client that no preparation is required

d. Withhold oral intake after midnight

Answer C is correct. The nurse should inform the client that no preparation is required for the *H. pylori* blood test. Answer A is incorrect because the nurse does not need to administer glucose prior to to the test. Answer B is incorrect because this step is associated with the preparation required for a breath test. Answer D is also incorrect because the client does not have to withhold oral intake prior to the blood test for *H. pylori*.

86. The nurse has been assigned to a client who was admitted to the unit after an abdominal cholecystectomy. When assessing the client's intake and outtake after 12 hours, the nurse recognizes that the the following finding needs to be reported to the doctor:

a. The 10mL output from the Jackson-Pratt drain

b. The absence of stool

c. The Foley catheter output of 285mL

d. The nasogastric tube output of 150mL

Answer C is correct. The nurse should report the

abnormal client's urinary output to the doctor. The normal urinary output is 30–50mL per hour. The client's urinary output is therefore below the normal range indicating the need for additional fluids. Answer A is incorrect because the output from the Jackson-Pratt drain is expected to be small. Answer B is incorrect because the client is also expected to not have a stool in the 12 hours following an abdominal cholecystectomy. Answer D is also incorrect because the output amount given is not excessive.

87. The client with symptoms of pseudomembranous colitis is admitted into the hospital. Which of the following symptoms indicates to the nurse that the client has contracted *Clostridium difficile*?

a. Anorexia, fever, and weight loss

b. Cough, fever, and shortness of breath

c. Diarrhea which contains mucus and blood

d. The client is developing ulcers on the lower extremities

Answer C is correct. This is because clients who have contracted *Clostridium difficile* often develop pseudomembranous colitis, the symptoms of which is the passage of diarrhea that contains white blood cells, mucus, and blood. Answers A, B, and D are incorrect because these symptoms are not specific to and infection with *Clostridium difficile*.

88. The client with cirrhosis and abdominal ascites has been admitted to the unit. The nurse knows to give the client snacks which are high in:

a. Fat

b. Potassium

c. Protein

d. Sodium

Answer C is correct. The nurse should provide the client with cirrhosis who has developed abdominal ascites with snacks that are high in protein because the client requires additional calories and protein. It is important to remember here however that the client's protein intake should be limited should the client's ammonia level increase. Answer A is incorrect because the client does not require any additional fat. Answer B is incorrect because the client's potassium intake need not be increased either. Answer D is also incorrect because the client should be placed on a diet that is low in sodium.

89. The nurse has been assigned to a client who is recovering from an episode of acute pancreatitis. Which of the following diets should the nurse include on the client's care plan?

a. A diet that is both high in protein and high in sodium

b. A high-carbohydrate and high-protein diet

c. A high-fat and low in sodium diet

d. A low-fat and low-protein diet

Answer D is correct. This is because clients who are recovering from acute pancreatitis should be placed on a diet which is both low in protein and low in fat. Answer A, B, and C are all incorrect because these diets are not suitable for the client.

90. The nurse is assessing a client with a duodenal ulcer who has been admitted to the hospital. Which of the following findings should the nurse immediately report to the physician?

a. BP 110/88, pulse 56

b. BP 82/60, pulse 130

c. Pulse 68, respirations 24

d. Pulse 82, respirations 16

Answer B is correct. The client is exhibiting both an increased pulse rate and a decreased blood pressure. These are both findings which are associated with shock and bleeding and which should be immediately reported to the physician. Answers A, C, and D are all incorrect because these findings are all normal and therefore not of concern.

91. The nurse is caring for a client with gastroesophageal reflux disease (GERD). Which of the following instructions should the nurse include on the

client's discharge plan?

a. Avoid carbonated beverages

b. Eat lemons and oranges as a healthy snack

c. Sleep on your right side only

d. Try and eat small snacks before bedtime

Answer A is correct. The client should be instructed to avoid carbonated beverages. This is because these beverages the incidence of gastroesophageal reflux by increasing the pressure in the stomach. Answer B is incorrect because clients with GERD should avoid acidic and spicy foods and beverages. This is because these irritate the gastric mucosa. Answer C is incorrect because the client should be instructed to sleep on the left side. Answer D is also incorrect because the client should avoid eating 3-4 hours before bedtime.

92. The client with bleeding from the upper gastrointestinal system has been admitted into the nurse's care. The nurse expects the client's stools to be which of the following?

a. Black

b. Brown

c. Clay-colored

d. Green

Answer A is correct. This is because one of the symptoms of upper gastrointestinal bleeding are stools which are black or tarry. Answer B is incorrect because normal stools are brown-colored. Answer C is incorrect because clay-colored stool is a symptom related to biliary obstruction. Answer D is also incorrect because green stool is associated with large amounts of bile or infection.

93. The nurse preparing a client with peritoneal dialysis for discharge. The nurse should instruct the client to notify the physician immediately if:

a. The client experiences a feeling of fullness when the dialysate is instilled

b. The client notices a tugging sensation as the dialysate drains

c. The dialysate returns appear to be cloudy

d. The dialysate returns are slower than usual

Answer C is correct. The client should be instructed to immediately notify his physician if the dialysate returns appear to be whitish or cloudy. This is because this could be a sign of infection and impending peritonitis. Answer A, B, and D are all incorrect because these are all expected and the client therefore does not need to notify the clinic.

94. The nurse has been assigned to a client with duodenal ulcers. Which of the following symptoms can the nurse expect the client to exhibit?

a. Epigastric pain after meals

b. Frequent bouts of diarrhea

c. Presence of blood in the client's stools

d. Vomiting shortly following meals

Answer C is correct. This is because melena, or blood in the stool, is a symptom that is common clients with duodenal ulcers. Answers A and D are incorrect because these are symptoms which are associated with gastric ulcers. Answer B is also incorrect because diarrhea is not a symptom associated with duodenal ulcers.

95. The physician has ordered Versed (midazolam) for a client who has been scheduled for a colonoscopy. The nurse knows that the client will:

a. Be able to remember the procedure within 2–3 days

b. Be able to remember the procedure within 2–3 hours

c. Not be able to remember the procedure

d. Not be able to remember what happened before the procedure

Answer C is correct. The nurse knows that the client who received Versed, a medication which produces conscious sedation, will not remember having the procedure done at all. Answers A, B, and D are all incorrect because these are all inaccurate statements.

96. The nurse has been assigned to a client with hepatitis C who has been scheduled for a liver biopsy. Which of the following should the nurse include on the client's teaching plan?

a. After the procedure, cleansing enemas should be given every morning

b. Blood coagulation studies might be done before the procedure

c. The nurse should inform the client that the procedure is noninvasive and causes no pain

d. The nurse should instruct the client to lie on the left side after the biopsy

Answer B is correct. Due to the risk of bleeding during a liver biopsy, laboratory tests are done before the procedure in order to find out whether the client has any problems with coagulation. Answer A is incorrect because no enemas are given. Answer C is incorrect because the procedure is invasive and does cause some pain. Answer D is also incorrect because the client needs to lie on the right side after the biopsy.

97. The client with cirrhosis of the liver has been admitted to the unit. Which is of the following is most helpful in helping the nurse determine whether the client has ascites?

a. A bimanual palpation for hepatomegaly

b. An assessment for a fluid wave

c. An inspection of the abdomen for enlargement

d. Daily measurement of abdominal girth

Answer D is correct. Measuring the abdominal girth on a daily basis is the most accurate and most specific way in which the nurse can detect any changes in the size of the client's abdomen. Answers A, B, and C are incorrect because they are not the best way in which the nurse can determine whether ascites is present.

98. The nurse is caring for a client with cirrhosis. The nurse notices that the client has developed signs of heptorenal syndrome. Which of the following diets should the nurse encourage?

a. A diet which is high in carbohydrate which is high in sodium

b. A diet which is high protein with moderate sodium

c. A low-carbohydrate diet which is also high protein

d. A low-protein, low-sodium diet

Answer D is correct. In order to decrease serum ammonia levels, clients who exhibit signs of heptorenal syndrome should be placed on a low-protein, low-sodium diet. Answer A is incorrect because although a high-carbohydrate diet would supply the client with calories, a high sodium intake would not be appropriate. Answer B is incorrect because sodium intake should be restricted and because the client will not benefit from a diet which is high in protein. Answer C is also incorrect because sodium should be restricted and because a diet which is high in protein will only serve to increase the client's ammonia levels. The client should therefore limit both sodium and protein intake.

99. The nurse is preparing a client with gastrointestinal disorder who has been prescribed a gluten-free diet for discharge. Which of the following diet choices would indicate to the nurse that the client has well understood the discharge instructions?

a. Bran cereal

b. Chocolate chip cookies

c. Steamed broccoli

d. Wheat toast

Answer C is correct. This food choice would indicate to the nurse that the client has understood the teaching plan. This is because fruits and fresh vegetables can be included on a gluten-free diet. Answers A, B, and D are all incorrect because all these food choices contain gluten.

100. The nurse is caring for a client with end stage renal disease who has been maintained with peritoneal dialysis. Which of the following instructions should the nurse give to the client if the dialysate return is slowed?

a. Alter your position and try turning from side to side

b. Gently retract the dialyzing catheter

c. Irrigate the dialyzing catheter with saline

d. You can skip the next scheduled infusion

Answer A is correct. If the dialysate return is slowed, the nurse should instruct the client to change his position or to try to move from side to side. This is because this should help improve the dialysate return. Answers B, C, and D are all incorrect because these are instructions which should be given to clients who are maintained on peritoneal dialysis.

101. The client with hepatitis C who has experienced cirrhosis changes in the past is admitted to the unit after a liver biopsy. The nurse knows to place the client into which of the following positions?

a. Left Sim's

b. Right side lying position

c. Supine

d. Trendelenburg

Answer B is correct. Clients who have undergone liver biopsies are at risk of developing hemorrhages. Because of this, the nurse should position the client on the right side in order to keep pressure on the area and prevent bleeding. Answers A, C, and D are all incorrect positions given the location of the liver.

102. The client with a possible bowel obstruction is admitted to the hospital. Which of the following questions would be most useful in helping the nurse

obtain information regarding the client's condition?

a. "Describe your usual diet to me."

b. "Have you noticed an increase in the size of your abdomen?"

c. "How would you describe the pain?"

d. "What does your vomit look like?"

Answer A is correct. This is because inquiring about the client's diet will be most helpful in identifying the problem and in obtaining information that could support the diagnosis. Answer B is helpful as swelling could be indicative of an obstruction. Answer C is helpful because pain is likely to decrease as the bowel obstruction progresses. Answer D is helpful because a description of the vomit could help the nurse identify the type of obstruction. In this scenario however, Answers B, C, and D are incorrect because Answer A is the most useful question.

The nurse has been assigned to a client with a suspected peptic ulcer. Which of the following exams would be most helpful in determining whether the diagnosis is correct?

A barium studies X-ray

A gastric analysis

An endoscopy procedure

An upper-gastrointestinal X-ray

Answer C is correct. All of the exam procedures above can be used to diagnose an ulcer. The endoscopic exam however, is the most accurate test and is therefore the correct answer. Answers A, B, and D are all incorrect because these exams are not as accurate.

Fluids and Electrolytes

Section 1: Introduction to Fluids and Electrolytes

Cells maintain a balance called homeostasis through constant transference of electrolytes and fluids in and out of cells. Fluid regulation is essential to homeostasis because alterations in electrolyte or water levels can cause many bodily functions to fail. Because of this and because of the large body fluid component, fluid balance is of prime importance in maintaining health – not only does body fluid assist in the effective transport of nutrients, gases and waste products around the body, but it also promotes body temperature regulation.

As a nurse, one of your main responsibilities is to assess the patient's fluid balance or imbalance. A loss of 20% of body fluid for example, can be fatal. Because of this, nurses play a pivotal role in the care and management of burn patients. By replacing the client's body fluid, the nurse can provide life-saving care.

The study of body fluid regulation and acid-base balance is one of the most difficult concepts to grasp. Because of this, it is important to spend enough time reviewing the care of clients with fluid, electrolyte, and acid-base imbalances in your preparation for the NCLEX. On top of this, it is also crucial to practice applying your knowledge with multiple practice questions. This concise preparation guide will cover the key points that you will need to know to be successful in the respiratory portion of your NCLEX test.

The guide begins with an outline of the topics and key facts on fluid, electrolyte, and acid-base imbalances that you need to remember for the exam. The list of subtopics can be seen on the contents page. In Section 3 of this guide you can apply and test your knowledge with over 100 topic-specific practice questions. All answers to the questions are given, along with detailed rationales for correct and incorrect answers to further your knowledge and understanding of the topic.

Remember that ambition is the first step to success. The second step is action – hard work and determination. Purchasing this guide is an indication of your ambition, now it's time to get to work!

Best wishes,

Eva Regan

Section 2: Fluid, Electrolyte and Acid-Base Imbalances Study Checklist

1. *Key Terms and Concepts*

Despite the fact that fluid and electrolyte balance and acid/base balance are separate in theory, they do directly relate to one another. For example, dehydration results in metabolic acidosis or a decrease in the pH. Overhydration on the other hand, results in metabolic alkalosis or an increase in the pH.

Before we dive into this topic, you will need to remember and have a good understanding of the following key terms:

- **Osmosis:** The process through which fluids and small particles move in and out of cells. This process transports hormones, nutrients, proteins, and other molecules into the cell and assist in the movement of waste products out of the cell for excretion by the body.

- **Filtration:** The process by which molecular particles are removed from the body fluid as they pass through semipermeable membranes.

- **Diffusion:** The process by which molecules move from a high concentration area to a low concentration area. Diffusion and active transport both allow anions and cations to pass in and out of the cell.

- **Active transport:** The process by which molecules can move from a low concentration area to a high concentration area.

- **Anions:** Negatively charged particles.

- **Cations:** Positively charged particles.

- **Electrolytes:** Particles that are either positively or negatively charged. Both anions and cations are electrolytes. Changes in pH are caused by the concentration of electrolytes.

- **pH:** A logarithmic measure of hydrogen ion concentration.

- **Acidosis:** An excessively acid condition of tissues and body fluids. Acidosis occurs when there is an accumulation of carbonic acid (H_2CO_3) and a decrease of bicarbonate hydrogen ions (HCO_3-).

- **Alkalosis:** An excessively alkaline condition of tissues and body fluids. Alkalosis occurs when there is an increase in bicarbonate hydrogen ions (HCO_3-) and there is a loss of carbonic acid (H_2CO_3).

2. *How the Body Regulates pH*

As a nurse, you will need to be able to evaluate pH in clients. To be able to do this, it is important to understand how the body regulates pH and the effect this has on the fluids and electrolytes inside the body.

- The ideal pH level of the body is 7.4 and a normal pH level ranges anywhere between 7.35 and 7.45.
- The body maintains its pH level by keeping the ratio of bicarbonate hydrogen ions (HCO_3-) to carbonic acid (H_2CO_3) at a 20:1 ratio.
- This relationship however, constantly changes and is only recovered thanks to our lungs and kidneys.
- Acidosis occurs when the body's pH falls below 7.40. It is considered to be an **uncompensated acidosis** when the pH falls below 7.35
- Alkalosis occurs when the body's pH rises above 7.40. it is considered to be an **uncompensated alkalosis** where the pH is above 7.45.

The body has two natural buffer systems that help to regulate the pH, thereby preventing acidosis and alkalosis from occurring:

- **The lungs:** The lungs retain and excrete carbonic acid in the form of carbon dioxide (CO_2).
- **The kidneys:** The kidneys assist in regulating pH by excreting or retaining sodium bicarbonate ($NaHCO_3$). They also do this by excreting both acidic and alkaline urine. The kidneys also help secret free $H+$ ions and by reabsorbing $NaHCO_3$.

Acidosis and alkalosis are both abnormal conditions that are typically caused by a condition or disease. In order to determine whether a client is in respiratory or metabolic acidosis or alkalosis, it is important to understand the normal blood gas values.

The normal PaCo2 blood gas value is 35-45 mm Hg. An abnormal PaCO2 with normal HCO3 indicates that the condition is **respiratory.**

- PaCO2 greater than 45 is indicative of respiratory acidosis
- PaCO2 below 35 is indicative of respiratory alkalosis

The normal HCO3 blood gas value is 22-26 mEq/L. An abnormal HCO3 with normal PaCO2 indicates that the condition is **metabolic.**

- HCO3 below 22 is indicative of metabolic acidosis
- HCO3 greater than 36 is indicative of metabolic alkalosis

It is important to remember these values for the exam. In the next section, we will discuss how these disorders can occur, the associated symptoms, and how a nurse should care for a client with acidosis or alkalosis.

3. *Caring for a Client with Acidosis*

Acidosis, the condition where there is too much acid in the body, is classified as either respiratory or metabolic acidosis.

Respiratory acidosis: pH down, CO2 up, HCO3 up

Respiratory acidosis occurs when there is accumulation of carbonic acid coupled and a lack of oxygenation. This results when the rate of ventilation decreases in relation to the amount of carbonic acid produced. This eventually leads to an accumulation of CO_2 that causes pH to fall below 7.35.

Common causes of respiratory acidosis include:

- **Acute lung conditions or diseases.**
- **Anesthesia or overuse of sedative drugs.** Note: There is a risk of narcotic overdose when a client has been administered anesthesia followed by a narcotic medication. Because of this, the nurse should also keep an antidote nearby, i.e. naloxone hydrochloride (Narcan).
- **Chest deformities or injuries.**
- **Chronic obstructive lung disease.**
- **Head injury.** The type of head injury that suppresses respirations.
- **Overbreathing of CO_2 for an extended duration.**
- **Paralysis of the respiratory muscles.**
- **Upper airway obstruction.**

A nurse should also know and be able to recognize the **symptoms of metabolic acidosis**. It is also important for you to remember these for the exam. They include:

- Dull sensorium
- Restlessness
- Apprehension
- Hypersomnolence
- Coma
- An increase in respiratory rate is an early symptom
- Perspiration
- An increase in the client's heart rate

- Hypoxia: Slow respirations and periods of apnea or Cheyne-Stokes respirations (breathing marked by periods of apnea lasting 10–60 seconds followed gradually by hyperventilation) are later symptoms that can result in cyanosis. Earlier signs of hypoxia include tachypnea and tachycardia.

In caring for a client with respiratory acidosis, the nurse should:

- Carefully check signs of respiratory distress
- Encourage fluids to thin secretions
- Perform chest physiotherapy
- Maintain a patent airway

Metabolic acidosis: pH down, CO2 down, HCO3 down

Metabolic acidosis happens when the pH falls below 7.40. This is triggered either by a loss of bicarbonate hydrogen ions (HCO3–) or a significant gain of carbonic acid (H2CO3). Common causes of metabolic acidosis include:

- **Anorexia:** Which causes cell starvation.
- **Certain disease states**: Disease states that lead to excessive metabolism of fats in the absence of usable carbohydrates - can result in a rise of ketoacids.
- **Diabetes mellitus:** A lack of usable insulin can lead to ketoacidosis and hyperglycemia.
- **Diarrhea**: Loss of HCO3 can lead to dehydration. Dehydration is a common cause for acidosis.

- **Excessive ingestion.**
- **Lactic acidosis**.
- **Overuse of diuretics**: In particular, overuse of non-potassium-sparing diuretics.
- **Sepsis or overwhelming infections:** Sepsis can lead to cell death and therefore an accumulation of nitrogenous waste.
- **Renal failure**: Renal failure can lead to the accumulation of waste in the body. —
- **Terminal stages of Addison's disease**: Adrenal insufficiency results in sodium and water loss which leads to a decrease in blood pressure and hypovolemic shock.

A nurse should also know and recognize the **symptoms of metabolic acidosis**, which include:

- A decrease in $PaCO_2$
- A decrease in pH
- A decreased serum CO_2
- An increase in potassium
- Anorexia
- Coma
- Diarrhea
- Drowsiness
- Fruity breath
- Headache
- Hyperventilation
- Increased acid in the urine
- Large volumes of dilute urine (polyuria)

- Lethargy
- Loss of consciousness
- Nausea
- Vomiting

Treating metabolic acidosis requires early diagnosis and treatment of the factors that are causing the condition. The following interventions are required to care for a client with metabolic acidosis:

- **Monitor the potassium level (K+) of the client and treat accordingly.**
    - **Hyperkalemia** describes the condition where the potassium level in the bloodstream is higher than normal.
    - Symptoms of hyperkalemia include nausea, malaise, diarrhea, muscle irritability, flaccid paralysis, and general weakness.
    - **Hypokalemia** describes the conditions when there is a deficiency of potassium in the blood.
    - Symptoms of hypokalemia include vomiting, shortness of breath, diminished reflexes, weak pulse, shallow respirations, and depressed U waves on the ECG.
    - Note: When administering potassium remember that it should be given with juice to counter the bitter taste. More importantly, remember to assess the client's renal function before administering potassium. Because the kidney assists in regulation potassium, if potassium is administered and the client has renal disease, this could lead to hyperkalemia which can be life-threatening.

- Monitor for any vital signs as to the quality of pulses, and intake and output.
- Diabetes should be treated with glucose for hypoglycemia and with insulin for hyperglycemia. Frequent blood glucose checks should be performed if the client is diabetic.
- Addison's diseases should be treated with cortisone preparations, fluids for shock, and a high sodium diet.
- Hypovolemia should be treated with blood transfusions, a volume expander, and a shock.
- Lactic acidosis should be treated with oxygen and NaHCO3.
- Renal failure should be treated with a transplant and diet changes or with dialysis.

4. *Caring for a Client with Alkalosis*

Alkalosis is the condition in which the body fluids contain excess base (alkali). There are different types of alkalosis: respiratory alkalosis and metabolic alkalosis.

Respiratory alkalosis: pH up, CO2 down, HCO3 down

Respiratory alkalosis is caused by low CO2 levels in the blood which can be caused by hyperventilation. Common causes of respiratory alkalosis include:

- Anxiety
- Being at a high altitude
- Hypoxia (or more generally, a lack of oxygen)

It is important for the nurse and nursing student sitting the NCLEX to be aware of the **symptoms of respiratory alkalosis** which include:

- A decrease in PaCO2
- An increase in pH
- Decreased levels of K+
- Deep, rapid respirations
- Fainting
- Fear
- Feelings of anxiety
- Hysteria
- Normal or decreased CO2 levels
- Numbness and a tingling sensation in the hands and feet
- Seizures
- Tetany

The following are the interventions a nurse should take when caring for a client with respiratory alkalosis. Firstly however, the nurse should determine what the cause for the hyperventilation is before taking the correct intervention.

- Using a re-breathing bag or breathing in a paper bag to facilitate retaining CO_2
- Decreasing the tidal volume and rate of ventilator settings

- Sedation
- Stress reduction

Metabolic alkalosis: pH up, CO2 up, HCO3 up

Metabolic alkalosis is caused by an accumulation of HCO3 or a loss of acid that causes the pH to rise above 7.45. Common causes of metabolic alkalosis include:

- Fistulas high in the gastrointestinal tract that can lead to a loss of hydrochloric acid
- Ingestion or retention of a base
- Steroid therapy or Cushing's syndrome (hypersecretion of cortisol) that can lead to sodium, hydrogen (H+) ions, and fluid retention
- Vomiting or nasogastric suction as this can also lead to loss of hydrochloric acid

It is also important for the nurse and nursing student to know and be able to recognize the **symptoms of metabolic alkalosis** which include:

- An increased NaHCO3
- Atrial tachycardia and depressed T waves associated with hypokalemia
- Attempts to retain CO2 resulting in slow, shallow respirations
- Diarrhea leading to a loss of hydrochloric acid

- Fidgeting and twitching tremors associated with hypokalemia or hyperkalemia
- Nausea
- Normal or increased CO2 levels
- pH levels above 7.45
- Vomiting

The following are the correct nursing intervention for treating clients with metabolic alkalosis:

- Administering potassium replacements
- Assessing for neurological changes
- Monitoring for dysrhythmias
- Monitoring intake and output

5. _How the Body Regulates Electrolytes_

Fluid in the body is compartmentalized into intercellular fluid and extracellular fluid.

- **Intracellular:** Two thirds of the fluid inside the body is intercellular. Intracellular fluid is fluid that is within the cell, i.e. within the vascular space. The major intracellular electrolytes are potassium and magnesium.
- **Extracellular:** One third of the fluid inside the body is extracellular. Extracellular fluid is fluid that is outside the cell, i.e. within the interstitial space. The major

extracellular electrolytes are sodium and chloride.

The distribution of body fluid inside the body is dependent on muscle mass and age. In an adult, the total body water is around 60% of the total body weight in kg. The total body water in infants and the elderly is around 70-80%. Because fatty tissue contains less water than muscle, infants and the elderly lose fluid at a faster rate compared to adults and therefore become dehydrated more quickly.

There are other health problems, directly relating to aging clients, the nurse should be aware of as these may upset the fluid, electrolyte and acid-base balance:

- Diabetes mellitus
- Liver disease
- Osteoporosis
- Poor appetite
- Renal failure

Electrolytes in the body are regulated by:

- **The endocrine system:** The endocrine system helps to keep sodium and potassium levels within the normal range by stimulating an antidiuretic hormone.

- **The gastrointestinal system:** This helps regulate gastric juices in the small bowl and in the stomach.

- **The vascular system:** The heart is what transports electrolytes in the blood.

- **The kidneys:** The kidney help regulate electrolytes through its glomeruli filter which filters out potassium and sodium (smaller particles) and by retaining protein (a larger particle).

6. *Know Your Lab Values!*

All fluid compartments in the body contain water and solutes or electrolytes. In order to care for clients with alternations in fluid and electrolytes, it is firstly important for a nurse to know the normal electrolyte values.

It is important to remember these normal lab values as they may be included in the NCLEX exam questions:

- **Total Serum Calcium (Ca+):** 8.5–10.5 mg/dL; 4.5–5.5 mEq/L
- **Serum Chloride (Cl–):** 95–105 mEq/L
- **Serum Magnesium (Mg+):** 1.5–2.5 mEq/L
- **Serum Phosphorus (P–):** 2.5–4.5 mEq/L
- **Serum Potassium (K+):** 3.5–5.5 mEq/L
- **Serum Sodium (Na+):** 135–145 mEq/L

Below are some other normal lab values that the nurse should remember and which will be of great help when evaluating fluids and electrolytes. Do note however that lab values fluctuate slightly depending on the age and gender of the client.

- **Carbon Dioxide Content:** 35-45 mEg/L
- **Serum Osmolality:** 280-295 mOsm/kg
- **Blood Urea Nitrogen (BUN):** 7-22 mg/dl
- **Serum Creatinine:** 6 – 1.35 mg/dl
- **Serum Glucose:** 70-110 mg/dl
- **Serum Albumin:** 3.5-5.5 g/dl
- **Urinary pH:** 4.5-8.0 mOsm/L
- **Hematocrit:** 44-52% (Male), 39-47% (Female)

Lastly, it is also important to note the following medications that can change electrolytes:

- Antacids
- Aspirin and NSAIDS
- Constipation
- Diuretics
- Lack of muscle mass
- Laxatives
- Osteoporosis
- Skin breakdown

7. _Diagnosing and Treating Clients with Electrolyte imbalances_

An alteration in electrolytes leads to a disequilibrium. In this section, we will talk about the causes and symptoms of alterations in electrolytes and how these can be treated. Firstly however, it is important to point out the diagnostic tests that are used to determine fluid and electrolyte and acid base balance. These include:

- Chest x-ray
- Serum levels for electrolytes
- Serum pH levels
- Sweat analysis
- Urinary lab values

Potassium imbalance

Potassium regulates protein synthesis, glycolysis, and glycogen synthesis. If cells become damaged, potassium leaves the cell, which can, depending on renal function, result in hyperkalemia or hypokalemia.

HYPERKALEMIA:

- **Causes:**
    - Addison's disease
    - Excessive use of salt substitutes
    - Potassium-sparing diuretics
    - Renal failure

- **Symptoms:**
    - Cramps
    - Diarrhea
    - EKG changes – peaked T waves, wide QRS complexes, or prolonged P-R intervals
    - Muscle twitching
    - Muscle weakness
    - Paresthesia
    - Slow pulse rate

- **Treatment:**
    - o Administer Calcium gluconate to protect the heart and decrease arrhythmias
    - o Administer sodium carbonate to counteract acidosis
    - o Dialysis, particularly if renal failure is present
    - o Give glucose and insulin to promote movement of potassium from the extracellular space back into the cells
    - o Monitor digitalis levels
    - o Monitor intake and output
    - o Monitor lab values
    - o Monitor serum potassium and EKG closely

HYPOKALEMIA:

- **Causes:**
    - o Medications such as digoxin, diuretics, and steroids

- **Symptoms:**
    - o Confusion
    - o Decreased specific gravity of the urine
    - o EKG changes – inverted T waves, depressed S-T segment
    - o Lethargy
    - o Nausea
    - o Vomiting
    - o Weak pulse

- **Treatment:**
    - o Change diet by increasing intake of foods high in potassium such as bananas, baked potatoes with the peel, dried fruit and melons

- o Change prescription to potassium-sparing diuretics
- o Check magnesium, chloride, and protein levels when replacing potassium
- o IV KCI on an IV pump or IV controller
- o Monitor input and output
- o Give potassium supplements. Before administering potassium however, the nurse should assess the client's renal function.
  - Administer oral liquid potassium with juice, such as orange or tomato juice to facilitate absorption of potassium.
  - If administering potassium IV, the nurse should dilute the potassium (as it can otherwise cause discomfort by burning the vein) and must always infuse using a controller because hyperkalemia can result in arrhythmias and death.

Sodium imbalance

Sodium maintains urine concentration, extracellular volume and acid-base balance. Along with potassium, it also promotes impulse transmission in nerves and muscle fibers. Diet is a major source of sodium. The minimum sodium requirement for an adult is 2 grams a day, although many consume far more sodium. Too much sodium results in hypernatremia. Too little sodium on the contrary, results in hyponatremia

HYPERNATREMIA:

- **Causes:**

- o Corticosteroids
- o Cushing's disease
- o Excessive sodium intake
- o Fever
- o Renal failure
- **Symptoms:**
  - o Agitation
  - o Confusion
  - o Decreased myocardial control
  - o Dry and flaky skin
  - o Reduced cardiac output
- **Treatment:**
  - o Administer diuretics
  - o Administer treatment for fever
  - o Correct water balance
  - o Decrease sodium content in diet
  - o Dialysis
  - o Monitor intake and output

HYPONATREMIA:

- **Causes:**
  - o Congestive heart failure
  - o Diuretics
  - o Hyperglycemia
  - o Renal disease
  - o Wound drainage

- **Symptoms:**
  - o Anorexia
  - o Decreased sensorium
  - o Decreased special gravity of urine
  - o Dry skin
  - o Headache
  - o Lethargy

o Mucous membranes
o Muscle weakness
o Oliguria
o Polyuria
o Rapid pulse

- **Treatment:**
  o Check complete blood count
  o Check urine specific gravity
  o Monitor intake and output
  o Replace sodium either by adding more to the diet or by IV therapy administration

Chloride imbalance

Chloride assists in the maintenance of acid-base balances and of osmotic pressure. It also promotes the formation of hydrochloric acid. Chloride is regulated by the gastrointestinal system and the kidneys and chloride intake comes mostly from the diet, in particular foods of high salt content. A higher than normal chloride level results in hyperchloremia, whereas chloride levels which are below the normal value lead to hypochloremia.

HYPERCHLOREMIA:

a. **Causes:**
o Increased consumption of salt

b. **Symptoms:**
o No specific symptoms other than those that can be associated with an excess of sodium

c. **Treatment:**
o Assess electrolytes
o Monitor intake and output
o Reduce salt intake in diet

HYPOCHLOREMIA:

d. **Causes:**
o Excessive infusion of hypotonic solutions
o Nasogastric suction
o Sodium deficiency
o Sodium loss through renal system
o Vomiting

e. **Symptoms:**
o No specific symptoms other than those that come with a loss of sodium

f. **Treatment:**
o Administer sodium and chloride
o Monitor for signs of acidosis

Calcium imbalance

Calcium assists with the strength and density of teeth and bones, muscle contractility, and normal clotting. Calcium is regulated by the renal system, the gastrointestinal system, and by Calcitonin; a thyroid hormone. A higher than normal calcium level results in hypercalcemia. Calcium levels which are below the normal value lead to hypocalcemia.

HYPERCALCEMIA:

- **Causes:**
    - Excessive calcium and vitamin D
    - Glucocorticoids
    - Hyperparathyroidism
    - Thiazide diuretics

- **Symptoms:**
    - Decreased clotting
    - Disorientation
    - EKG changes – shortened Q-T intervals
    - Hypertension
    - Hypotonic bowel sounds
    - Increased urinary output
    - Renal calculi
    - Tachycardia

- **Treatment:**
    - Assess for renal calculi
    - Check for digitalis intoxication
    - Check for metabolic alkalosis
    - Decrease intake of vitamin D and calcium
    - Stay hydrated

HYPOCALCEMIA

- **Causes:**
    - Celiac disease
    - Crohn's disease
    - End stage renal disease
    - Immobility
    - Lactose intolerance
    - Pancreatitis
    - Thyroidectomy

- **Symptoms:**
  - o An increased heart rate
  - o Anxiety
  - o Positive Chvostek's sign – this is done by tapping the facial nerve and checking for facial twitching
  - o Dental caries
  - o Dull skin
  - o EKG changes – prolonged S-T and Q-T intervals
  - o Fatigue
  - o Hyperactive deep tendon reflexes
  - o Osteoporosis
  - o Positive Trousseau's sign – this is done by applying a blood pressure cuff to the arm and checking for carpo-pedal spasms
  - o Psychosis
  - o Thinning hair

- **Treatment:**
  - o Administer calcium and vitamin D supplements
  - o Check for metabolic acidosis
  - o Have tracheostomy available should the client experience laryngeal spasms
  - o Monitor and evaluate EKG
  - o Seizure precautions

Phosphorus imbalance

Phosphorus assists in the formation and activation of ATP and in the activation of B complex. It also assists in cell development, bone and teeth development, CHO, fat and protein metabolism. A higher than normal level of phosphorus results in hyperphospatemia and a lower than normal phosphorus level can lead to hypophosphatemia.

HYPERSPHOSPHATEMIA:

- **Causes:**
    - o Decreased renal function
    - o Hyperparathyroidism
    - o Hypocalcemia
    - o Increased phosphorus intake

- **Symptoms:**
    - o Increased serum phosphorus levels
    - o Muscle spasm
    - o Positive Chvostek's sign
    - o Positive Trousseau's sign

- **Treatment:**
    - o Administer aluminium hydroxide or other phosphate-binding medications
    - o Administer calcium supplements
    - o Decrease diet intake of food containing phosphorus
    - o Hemodialysis
    - o Reduce intake of medications containing phosphorus

HYPOPHOSPHATEMIA:

- **Causes:**
    - o Aluminium or magnesium antacids
    - o Hyperglycemia
    - o Malnutrition

- **Symptoms:**
    - o Cardiomyopathy

- o Decreased deep tendon reflexes
- o Irritability
- o Shallow respiration

- **Treatment:**
  - o Assess calcium levels
  - o Change diet to increase phosphorus intake
  - o Give phospho soda
  - o Monitor and evaluate EKG
  - o Monitor for muscle weakness
  - o Perform neurological assessment

Magnesium imbalance

Magnesium helps with DNA synthesis, activation of ATP and B complex, and muscle contraction. It also contributes to vasodilation, activates intracellular enzymes in carbohydrates and assists with protein synthesis, cardiac and skeletal muscle cells. A magnesium level which is higher than the normal value leads to hypermagnesemia, whereas a lower than normal magnesium level results in hypomagnesemia.

HYPERMAGNESEMIA:

- **Causes:**
  - o Increased ingestion of magnesium
  - o Renal failure

- **Symptoms:**
  - o Bradycardia

o Diminished deep tendon reflexes
o Drowsiness
o Hypotension
o Lethargy
o Respiratory depression

- **Treatment:**
    o Administer calcium gluconate
    o Dialysis
    o Monitor deep tendon reflexes (DTRs) – absence
      of patella reflex indicates toxicity
    o Monitor intake and output on an hourly basis
    o Monitor level of consciousness (LOC)
    o Provide ventilator support

HYPOMAGNESEMIA:

- **Causes:**
    o Alcoholism
    o Celiac disease
    o Crohn's disease
    o Diarrhea
    o Food containing citrate
    o Malnutrition

- **Symptoms:**
    o An increase in blood pressure
    o Confusion
    o Dysrhythmias
    o Hyperreflexia
    o Positive Chovstek's sign
    o Positive Trousseau's sign

- **Treatment:**

o Administer magnesium – always check renal
function prior to magnesium administration
and if IV magnesium is given, the nurse should
always use a controller
o Monitor deep tendon reflexes (DTRs) – absence
of which indicates toxicity to magnesium
o Monitor magnesium levels on an hourly basis –
decreased respiration indicates toxicity to
magnesium

8. _Pharmacological Interventions to Treat Disorders of Fluid_
and Electrolyte Balance and Acid-Base Balance

A recurring nursing intervention that is important when
caring for clients with fluid and electrolyte disorders is
treatment through pharmacological intervention. The nurse
and nursing student need to be aware of the most common
side and adverse effects of these medications. The
medications used to treat fluid, electrolyte and acid-base
imbalances include:

Aluminium hydroxide (Amphoget):

o Liquid forms are more effective
o Tablets should be chewed and ingested with
half a glass of water

- **Action:**
o Neutralizes gastric acids

- **Side effects:**
o Constipation

o Decreased phosphorus

Calcium carbonate (Tums):

    o Liquid forms are more effective
    o Tablets should be chewed and ingested with half a glass of water

- **Action:**
  - o Elevates gastric pH
  - o Reduces pepsin activity

- **Side effects:**
  - o Constipation
  - o Hypercalcemia

Calcium gluconate:

    o Check for signs of calcium renal calculi

- **Action:**
  - o Used in the treatment of hypocalcemia and magnesium toxicity

- **Side effects:**
  - o Can cause constipation
  - o Can lead to Hypercalcemia

Magaldrate (Riopan):

    o During the treatment, the nurse should monitor the client's magnesium levels

- **Action:**
  - o Neutralizes gastric acid

- **Side effects:**
  - Can cause diarrhea
  - Increases magnesium levels

MgSO4:

  - Insert Foley catheter
  - If administered IV, a controller should be used and titrate dosage
  - Monitor intake and output every hour
  - Monitor for toxicity – check for hypotension, oliguria, decreased respiration and absence of knee jerk reflex

- **Action:**
  - Used in the treatment of hypomagnesemia

- **Side effects:**
  - Diarrhea
  - Hot flashes

Potassium chloride:

  - Check client's renal function before administering
  - If oral liquid potassium is administered, give with juice for better absorption.
  - If potassium if administered IV, it should be diluted and an IV controller must be used for infusion.

- **Action:**
  - Used in the treatment of hypokalemia

- **Side effects:**

o Liquid potassium is bitter
o Irritating to the vein
o Can cause cardiac arrhythmias
o Can cause muscle spasms

Sodium bicarbonate:

o During the treatment, the nurse should monitor blood pH

- **Action:**
  o It acts as a systemic and local alkalizer

- **Side effects:**
  o Can cause alkalosis
  o Can lead to acid rebound

Section 3: Fluids and Electrolytes Practice Questions and Rationales

1. The client is being assessed for risk of hyperphosphatemia. Which of the following is most important for the nurse to obtain?

a. A history of minimal physical activity
b. A history of radiation treatment in the neck region
c. A history of the client's food intake
d. Any history of recent orthopedic surgery

Answer B is correct. This is because any radiation treatment to the neck could have damaged the parathyroid glands, which are located on the thyroid gland. This could interfere with calcium and phosphorus regulation. Answers A and C are incorrect because these are related to calcium regulation, not phosphorus regulation. Answers D is incorrect because it bears no relation to the question.

2. A client with cancer has been admitted to the oncology unit. Laboratory values reveal WBC 6500, Na+ 138, K+ 2.1, Hgb 12.6, uric acid 7.0, and platelets 192,000. The nurse assesses these findings as which of the following?

a. Myelosuppression
b. Leukocytosis
c. Hypokalemia

d. Hypernatremia

Answer C is correct. All lab results but apart from potassium are normal. The normal serum potassium value ranges between 3.5–5.5 mEq/L. A potassium level of 2.1 therefore indicates hypokalemia. Answers A, B, and D are incorrect because these values are all normal.

3. The client with hypokalemia is admitted for administration of an IV of normal saline to be infused at 80 ml/hour with 10 meq of KCl/hour. Before starting the infusion, it is crucial for the nurse to:

a. Asses the magnesium level
b. Assess the calcium level
c. Assess the creatinine level
d. Assess the sodium level

Answer C is correct. This is because prior to receiving potassium, it is important that the client is evaluated for renal function because the kidneys are the primary regulator of potassium. Answers A, B, and D are incorrect because it is not necessary to assess magnesium, calcium or sodium levels prior to administering potassium.

4. A client is admitted to the hospital. Laboratory values reveal a pH of 7.30, a HCO3 of 30, and a PaCO2 of

48mm Hg. Which of the following is the client experiencing?

a. Respiratory alkalosis

b. Respiratory acidosis

c. Metabolic alkalosis

d. Metabolic acidosis

Answer B is correct. The nurse should always assess the pH when checking arterial blood gases. The pH in this scenario is low. This is the first conclusion the nurse should make. Upon assessing the PaCO2 and HCO3, the nurse should find that both values are elevated in this case. The nurse can therefore evaluate that the client is experiencing respiratory acidosis. Answers A, C, and D are incorrect because the options given are inconsistent with the laboratory values.

5. The client with diabetes mellitus has been diagnosed with metabolic acidosis. Findings reveal a blood glucose level of 250 mg/dl. Which of the following symptoms is most commonly associated with ketoacidosis?

a. Tremors
b. Polydipsia

c. Perspiration

d. Oliguria

Answer B is correct. The client's blood glucose level is above normal, which is an indication that he is experiencing hyperglycemia, the symptoms of which are are polyuria, polydipsia, and polyphagia. On top of this, the client will also have a decreased sensorium and tachypnea. Answers A, B, and D are all incorrect because these are symptoms of hypoglycaemia.

6. The client with Cushing's disease will most likely exhibit symptoms of:

a. Hypermagnesemia

b. Hypernatremia

c. Hypocalcaemia

d. Hypokalemia

Answer B is correct. This is because clients with Cushing's disease have overactive adrenal glands and retain sodium and water. Answers A, C, and D are incorrect because they do not typically retain magnesium or lose calcium or potassium.

7. A client with cancer and metastasis to the bone is admitted to the unit. Which symptom of hypercalcemia

should the nurse be most concerned about?

a. Anorexia
b. Cardiac changes
c. Flaccid muscles
d. Weakness

Answer B is correct. This is because clients with hypercalcemia can have dysrhythmias (heart block), which can be life threatening. Answers A, C, and D are incorrect because monitoring cardiac changes should be given priority over the other symptoms listed.

8. When administering magnesium sulphate, which piece of equipment should be obtained for safety reasons?

a. A blood administration set

b. A wall suction device

c. An internal fetal heart monitor

d. An IV rate controller

Answer D is correct. If magnesium sulfate is administered too rapidly, it can become toxic and lead to respiratory arrest. Because of this, the nurse must always obtain an IV rate controller in order to ensure safe administration of magnesium sulfate. Answer A is incorrect because a standard IV administration set should be used. Answer B is incorrect because when administering magnesium sulfate, a wall suction device is not required. Answer C is also incorrect because an internal fetal monitor does not need to be inserted when administering magnesium sulfate. When the client is pregnant however, an external fetal monitor should be used.

9. A client admitted to the hospital complaints of shortness of breath. An unconfirmed diagnosis of respiratory acidosis is made. Which of the following sets of findings would support this diagnosis?

a. CO_2 of 30, HCO_3 of 22, pH of 7.34
b. CO_2 of 32, HCO_3 of 25, pH of 7.44
c. CO_2 of 45, HCO_3 of 26, pH of 7.45
d. CO_2 of 46, HCO_3 of 27, pH of 7.35

Answer D is correct. This is because a client with respiratory acidosis will have a lower than normal pH level. CO_2 excretion would also have increased due to respiratory problems. Like the findings show, there would also be an increase in HCO_3 because the kidneys are the compensating organ. Answer A is incorrect because it is metabolic acidosis. Answer B is incorrect because it is compensated alkalosis. And Answer C is likewise incorrect because it is alkalosis.

10. The client has been complaining of nausea and vomiting for the past three days. The physician has prescribed D51/2NS with potassium added. Which nursing intervention is most appropriate in this case?

a. Check the client's vital signs hourly

b. Check the sodium level

c. Obtain an 18-gauge cathlon to begin the infusion

d. Obtain an IV controller

Answer D is correct. Whenever potassium is added to IV fluids, an IV controller must be used under all circumstances due to the risk of cardiac arrhythmias arising from infusions that are too rapid. Answer A is incorrect because no data exists to say that hourly vital signs should be monitored. Answer B is incorrect because the client has a prescription for D51/2NS (which is the same in saline as the normal sodium level of the client). Answer C is likewise incorrect because the nurse can use any size cathlon for infusion. Obtaining an 18-gauge cathlon is not necessary.

11. The client with a blood glucose level of 545 mg/dl is admitted to the hospital. Which of the following actions should the nurse take?

a. The nurse inserts a Foley catheter

b. The nurse obtains NPH insulin for administration

c. The nurse prepares an IV of D10W

d. The nurse prepares to administer insulin IV

Answer D is correct. The nurse should order an IV with insulin because the client with blood glucose of 545 mg/dl is in metabolic acidosis. Answer A is incorrect because a Foley catheter is not necessary, although it may be ordered. Answer B is incorrect because the effect of D10W is to increase the client's glucose level which only serves to heighten the effect of his condition. Answer C is also incorrect because insulin will be ordered which is long-acting.

12. A client with a potassium level of 2.4 meq/L is admitted to the hospital. Which of the following symptoms should the nurse expect to see?

a. Muscle rigidity
b. Peaked T waves
c. Rapid respirations
d. U waves

Answer D is correct. Answer A is incorrect because the client's muscles will be flaccid when in hypokalemia.

Answer B is incorrect because peaked T waves indicate a potassium level which is higher than the normal value. Answer C is also incorrect because respirations will not be rapid but shallow.

13. A client with preeclampsia is admitted to the labor and delivery unit. An IV of magnesium sulfate is administrated per pump. Which of the following would indicate hypermagnesemia?

Absence of the knee-jerk reflex
Blood pressure of 150/80
Respirations of 30 per minute
Urinary output of 60 ml per hour

Answer A is correct. This is because the symptoms of toxicity to magnesium include an absence to the deep tendon reflexes. Other signs of toxicity include respirations under 12 per minute and oliguria. Answer B is incorrect because blood pressure in the above is within the normal range. Answer C is incorrect because if respirations fall below 12, oxygen support should be provided and infusion should be discontinued. Answer D is likewise incorrect because the urinary output here is also within the normal range. The nurse should further evaluate toxicity if the urinary output falls below 30ml per minute.

14. The client with anorexia nervosa is admitted to the hospital. The nurse should expect the client to show signs of which of the following conditions?

a. Metabolic acidosis

b. Metabolic alkalosis

c. Respiratory acidosis

d. Respiratory alkalosis

Answer A is correct. This is because clients with anorexia nervosa are in a state of negative nitrogen balance and are therefore most probably experiencing metabolic acidosis. Answer B is incorrect because clients with anorexia nervosa will have a deficit in HCO3 and an indication of the presence of metabolic alkalosis is an increase in HCO3. Answers C and D are incorrect because anorexia nervosa is a metabolic (and not a respiratory) disorder.

15. The client with hyperparathyroidism will have symptoms of:

a. Hypercalcemia
b. Hyperphosphatemia
c. Hypokalemia

d. Hyponatremia

Answer A is correct. Clients with hyperparathyroidism will have hypercalcemia and hypophosphatemia. This is because calcium is pulled from the bone into the serum of the body that increases calcium levels. Clients with hyperparathyroidism will often also have osteoporosis and renal calculi. Answers B, C, and D are incorrect because they will not have hyperphosphatemia, hypokalemia, or hyponatremia.

16. The nurse is caring for a client with metabolic acidosis associated with diabetes mellitus. A lab finding indicates blood glucose of 250 mg/dl. Which of the following symptoms will most likely accompany ketoacidosis?

a. Oliguria
b. Perspiration
c. Polydipsia
d. Tremors

Answer C is correct. The client's blood glucose level is above the normal value which means that they are in hyperglycemia, the symptoms of which include polydipsia, polyuria, and polyphagia. On top of this, the client will also experience a decrease in tachypnea and sensorium. Answers A, B, and D are all incorrect because these are symptoms of hypoglycemia.

17. A client with renal failure is admitted to the unit. Which of the following should be removed from the tray of the client?

a. Baked potato
b. Bread
c. Marshmallows
d. Peach

Answer A is correct. Because a client with renal failure should only receive limited amounts potassium, baked potatoes should be avoided because potato skin contains large amounts of potassium. Answers B and C are incorrect because these contain only limited amounts of potassium. Answer D is likewise incorrect. Although peaches contain some potassium, it doesn't contain as much as the baked potato.

18. The function of the lungs in acid-base balance is to perform which of the following actions?

a. Control HCO3 levels

b. Maintain sodium levels

c. Regulate potassium levels

d. Retain or blow off CO2

Answer D is correct. This is because by regulating the amount of CO2 that is exhaled or retained, the lungs help regulate acid-base balance in the body. Answers A, B, and C are incorrect because the lungs do not play any role in the regulation of HCO3 levels, sodium, or potassium levels.

19. The client with hypoparathyroidism who was admitted to the unit has a lack of parathyroid hormone. The client will most likely receive an administration for serum calcium level of which of the following values?

a. 3.5 mg/dl

b. 10.9 mg/dl

c. 14.7 mg/dl

d. 18.5 mg/dl

Answer A is correct. This is because the normal calcium level is 8.5–10.5 mg/dl. Answers B, C, and D are all incorrect because all of these findings would result in an above-normal value.

20. The client who had a motorcycle accident is admitted to the hospital and is likely to have extensive internal bleeding. The serum pH is 7.0, HCO3 is 20 mEq/dl, and the PaCO2 is 32 mm/Hg. The nurse should check the lab finding for which of the following conditions?

a. Metabolic acidosis

b. Metabolic alkalosis

c. Respiratory acidosis

d. Respiratory alkalosis

Answer A is correct. The client who has suffered internal bleeding will most likely be in metabolic acidosis. The lab findings support this – ph down, HCO3 down, PaCO2 down. Answers B, C, and D are incorrect because these are inconsistent with the laboratory values.

21. The nurse is responsible for instructing the client who lacks magnesium regarding dietary choices. Which food is a good source of magnesium?

a. Apple
b. Liver
c. Spinach
d. Squash

Answer C is correct. This is because spinach and other dark green vegetables provide a great source of magnesium. Answers A, B, and D are incorrect because these do not provide significant sources of magnesium.

22. An 80-year-old client with a temperature of 100.2°, urinary specific gravity of 1.032, and a dry tongue is admitted to the hospital. The nurse should anticipate an order prescription for:

a. A diuretic

b. An analgesic

c. An antibiotic

d. An IV of normal saline

Answer D is correct. This is because the client is most likely to be hyponatremic and hypovolemic. The high temperature and dry tongue can both be related to dehydration and the urinary specific gravity shows urinary concentration. Answers A, B, and C are incorrect because there isn't enough data to show that a diuretic, an analgesic or an antibiotic is necessary in this case.

23. A client with a serum calcium level of 10.0 mg/dL, a potassium level of 3.9 mEq/L, a blood glucose level of 98 mg/dL, and a blood urea nitrogen level of 30 mg/dL

has been admitted to the unit. Which of these values should the nurse immediately report to the doctor?

The blood glucose level of 98 mg/dL

The blood urea nitrogen level of 30 mg/dL

The potassium level of 3.9 mEq/L

The serum calcium level of 10.0 mg/dL

Answer B is correct. Answers A, C, and D are all incorrect because these levels are within the normal values.

24. The nurse is caring for several clients at the same time. Which of the following clients should receive priority of care?

a. A 35-year-old client with chest tubes and a CO_2 level of 48mE/L who has been in a motor vehicle accident

b. A female client with cirrhosis of the liver and a blood urea nitrogen level of 35mg/dl

c. An elderly client with an oxygen saturation level of 82% and emphysema

d. An elderly diabetic with a blood glucose level of 430 mg/dl

Answer D is correct. The client with a blood glucose of 430 mg/dl has priority of care because this client is at risk for diabetic coma. Answers A, B, and C are all incorrect. Changes in CO_2 level, BUN and oxygen saturation are all expected and therefore do not require priority of care.

25. The client with hypokalemia has a prescription for potassium that is to be administered orally. Before administering the potassium, the nurse should:

a. Insert a nasogastric tube

b. Monitor the client's creatinine level

c. Obtain milk to give the oral potassium

d. Request to order an ECG from the physician

Answer B is correct. Before administering potassium, the nurse should always assess the client's renal function. Renal function can be assessed by evaluating the client's creatinine level. The doctor should always be notified prior to potassium administration should the client have elevated creatinine levels (the normal creatinine laboratory value is .60–1.60 mg/dL). Answer A is incorrect because inserting a nasogastric tube in this case is necessary. Answer C is incorrect because potassium should be given with fruit juice and not with milk. Answer D is likewise incorrect because there is no need to request an ECG order from the doctor.

26. A client with hypokalemia has been admitted to the unit. The nurse is preparing to administer potassium. Which of the following is the best liquid for the nurse to dilute the potassium in?

a. Chocolate milk

b. Cranberry juice

c. Prune juice

d. Tomato juice

Answer B is correct. To facilitate absorption, potassium should be given in a juice which contains ascorbic acid. Tomato juice is the juice with the most ascorbic acid and is therefore very suitable for potassium administration. Other juices which can be used for this purpose include orange juice, grape juice, and pineapple juice. Answer A is incorrect because chocolate milk does not contain much ascorbic acid. Answers C and D are also incorrect because both cranberry and prune juice are less acidic and therefore less suitable.

27. The client with hypoparathyroidism is admitted to the unit. Findings indicate a calcium level of 7.6 mg/dL. Which of the following should the nurse anticipate to receive an order for?

a. Furosemide (Lasix)

b. Levothyroxin (Synthyroid)

c. Propanolol (inderal)

d. PTH (Forteo)

Answer D is correct. This is because the client with hypoparathyroidism will require supplementation with parathyroid hormone. Answers A, B, and C are all incorrect because these drugs are not used to treat clients with hypoparathyroidism.

28. The nurse is caring for a client with a magnesium level of 10.0 mEq/L. Which of the following indicates that the client has a toxic level of magnesium?

a. Deep tendon reflexes of 2+

b. Hot flashes

c. Respirations of 10 per minute

d. Urinary output of 40 mL per hour

Answer C is correct. This is because decreased respiration of fewer than 12 per minute, oliguria, and an absence of deep tendon reflexes are all signs of toxicity to magnesium. Answer A is incorrect because deep tendon reflexes of 2+ is a normal value. Answer B is incorrect because hot flashes are an expected side effect. And answer d is likewise incorrect a urinary output of 40 mL per hour is within the lower limits of the normal value.

29. Which of the following staff members should not be assigned to a client receiving magnesium intravenously?

a. The graduate registered nurse

b. The licensed practical nurse

c. The nursing assistant

d. The surgical resident

Answer C is correct. The nursing assistant should not be assigned to care for the client in this case. This is because magnesium can cause apnea and renal failure and apnea. Answer A is incorrect because a graduate registered nurse can report abnormalities and evaluate respiratory status and renal function. Answer B is incorrect because a licensed practical nurse can report alternations in renal function to the registered nurse, as well as evaluate urinary output. Answer D is also incorrect because a surgical resident would have finished medical school to further their career as a surgeon.

30. Which of the following should be kept ready when intravenous magnesium is to be administered?

a. Aminocaproic acid

b. AquaMEPHYTON

c. Calcium gluconate

d. Protamine sulfate

Answer C is correct. This is because calcium gluconate is the antidote for magnesium sulfate. Answer A is incorrect because Aminocaproic cid (Amicar) is the antidote for streptokinase. Answer B is incorrect because AquaMEPHYTON (Vitamin K) is the antidote for Coumadin (Sodium warfarin). Answer D is likewise incorrect because Protamine sulfate is the antidote for Heparin.

31. The client with a pH of 7.48, a CO2 level of 48 mEq/L, and a HCO3 level of 34 mEq/L is admitted to the unit. The nurse is aware that these laboratory values reveal:

a. Respiratory alkalosis

b. Respiratory acidosis

c. Metabolic alkalosis

d. Metabolic acidosis

Answer A is correct. All findings indicate that the client is in metabolic alkalosis. Answers B, C, and D are all incorrect because these are incorrect assessments of the given laboratory values.

32. The nurse assigned to a client receiving magnesium sulfate must carefully monitor the client for side effects associated with the medication therapy. Which side effect of magnesium sulfate should the nurse should expect to see?

a. Hypersomnolence

b. Decreased urinary output

c. Decreased respiratory rate

d. Absence of the knee jerk reflex

Answer A is correct. Sleepiness, lethargy and hot flashes are all expected side effects of magnesium sulfate. Answers B, C, and D are incorrect because decreased urinary output, decreased respiratory rate and an absence of the knee jerk reflect are all signs of toxicity and are therefore not among the expected side effects of the medication.

33. The nurse is assessing a client who has been placed on Digoxin (digitalis). Which of the following findings should the nurse report to the physician?

a. Chloride level of 98 mEq/L

b. Magnesium level of 1.8 mEq/L

c. Potassium level of 3.0 mEq/L

d. Sodium level of 138 mEq/L

Answer C is correct. This is because a potassium level of 3.0 is below the normal value. Answers A, B, and D are all incorrect because these are values within normal limits.

34. The physician ordered a low-potassium diet for the client with renal disease. Which of the following is highest in potassium?

a. Cake

b. Marshmallows

c. Mashed potatoes

d. Raisins

Answer D is correct. This is because dried fruits such as raisins are high in potassium. Answers A, B, and C are incorrect because these contain lower amounts of potassium.

35. The client with hypertension and renal disease has been admitted to the unit. Findings indicate a blood pressure of 190/100. The doctor decides to prescribe a potassium-sparing diuretic and a beta blocker. Which diuretic can the nurse expect an order for?

a. Torsemide (Demadex)

b. Spironolactone (Aldactone)

c. Hydrochlorothiazide (HTCZ)

d. Furosemide (Lasix)

Answer B is correct. This is because ALdactone is the only potassium-sparing diuretic among the ones given. Answers A, C, and D are all incorrect because they are not potassium-sparing diuretics.

36. The nurse is caring for a client with chronic obstructive pulmonary disease. Findings indicate a pH of 7.32, a CO2 level of 49 mEq/L and a HCO3 level is 26 mEq/L. Which of the following is the correct diagnosis?

a. Respiratory alkalosis

b. Respiratory acidosis

c. Metabolic alkalosis

d. Metabolic acidosis

Answer B is correct. The findings (low pH value, and elevated HCO3 and CO2 values) indicate that the client is in respiratory acidosis. Answers A, C, and D are incorrect for the same reason.

37. The nurse has been assigned a patient with ulcerative colitis. The nurse should prioritize care for which of the following is findings?

a. Anxiety

b. Fluid volume deficit

c. Impaired skin integrity

d. Nutrient alterations

Answer B is correct. This is because fluid volume deficit can result in metabolic acidosis and electrolyte loss. It should therefore be a priority on the care plan. Answers A, C, and D are incorrect because these are of lesser priority.

38. The client with Cushing's disease is admitted to the unit. The nurse knows that clients with an adrenal disorder such as Cushing's disease will most likely exhibit signs of which of the following conditions?

a. Hypercalcemia

b. Hyperkalemia

c. Hypermagnesemia

d. Hypernatremia

Answer D is correct. The client is most likely to exhibit signs of hypernatremia because clients with Cushing's disease often retain sodium. Answers A, B, and C are incorrect because signs of hypercalcemia, hyperkalemia, and hypermagnesemia are significantly less likely in the client with Cushing's disease.

39. The client with diabetes insipidus is admitted to the hospital. Which of the following findings supports this diagnosis?

a. Glucose of 110 mg/dL

b. Potassium of 3.8 mEq/dL

c. Sodium of 140 mEq/L

d. Specific gravity of 1.000

Answer D is correct. This is because the specific gravity given is low (the normal value ranges between 1.010 and 1.030). Clients with diabetes insipidus exhibit a lack of antidiuretic hormone, which results in a large volume of urinary output with a low specific gravity. Answers A, B, and C are all incorrect because these values are within their normal limits and are not directly associated with diabetes insipidus.

40. The nurse is assessing the history of an elderly client. Which statement made by the client might indicate a possible fluid and electrolyte imbalance?

a. "I drink a lot of ice tea."

b. "I regularly use a laxative for constipation."

c. "I sometimes have problems with dribbling urine."

d. "My skin is always so dry."

Answer B is correct. This is because the frequent use of laxatives can result in diarrhea and consequently electrolyte loss. Answers A, C, and D are incorrect because they are not of significance in this case.

41. The nurse has been assigned to a client with cancer. Laboratory values reveal the following findings: Hgb 12.6, WBC 6500, K+ 1.9, uric acid 7.0, Na+ 136, and platelets 178,000. The nurse assesses these findings as which of the following?

a. Hypernatremia

b Hypokalemia

c. Leukocytosis

d. Myelosuppression

Answer B is correct. From the findings given, the nurse can evaluate that the client is experiencing hypokalemia. Answers A, C, and D are incorrect because all these values are normal.

42. A client with a serum sodium of 170meq/L is admitted to the acute care unit. Which of the following behavior changes should ne nurse expect?

a. Anger

b. Depression

c. Mania

d. Psychosis

Answer C is correct. This is because the client has hypernatremia, a symptom of which is manic behavior. Answers A, B, and D are incorrect as these are not related to hypernatremia.

43. The 73-year-old client with hypomagnesemia is admitted. The physician ordered for magnesium sulfate. Which of the following actions by the nurse indicates an understanding of magnesium sulfate and its effects?

a. The nurse darkens the room

b. The nurse monitors the urinary output on an hourly basis

c. The nurse places a padded tongue blade near the client's bed

d. The nurse places a sign over the client's bed not to check blood pressures in the left arm

Answer B is correct. This is because the client who has been placed on magnesium sulfate should have a Foley catheter in place. Urinary output should be measured on an hourly bases and because oliguria is a sign of toxicity to magnesium sulfate. Answer A is incorrect because darkening the room will not help prevent toxicity. Answer C is incorrect because although a padded tongue blade should be kept on the side of the bed in case of a seizure, this has no relation to the magnesium sulfate infusion. Answer D is likewise incorrect because there is no need to refrain from checking the client's blood pressure in the left arm.

44. The nurse is caring for a client with hypomagnesemia. In order to assess the client's deep tendon reflexes which method should the nurse use to obtain the biceps reflex?

a. The nurse should instruct the client to dangle their legs as the nurse strikes the area below the patella with the blunt side of the reflex hammer

b. The nurse should instruct the client to place their arms loosely at their side as the nurse strikes the muscle insert just above the wrist

c. The nurse should place her thumb on the muscle inset in the antecubital space and taps the thumb briskly with the reflex hammer

d. The nurse should suspend the client's arm in an open hand while tapping the back of the client's elbow

Answer C is correct. This is because only the method described in answer C elicits different reflexes. Answer A is incorrect because this elicits the patella reflex. Answer B is incorrect because this elicits the radial nerve. Answer D is also incorrect because this elicits the triceps reflex.

45. A client with second-degree burns to the head, face, and neck is admitted to the hospital 2 hours after the injury occurred. Which of the following should the nurse be most concerned about?

a. Hyperkalemia

b. Hypernatremia

c. Hypovolemia

d. Laryngeal edema

Answer D is correct. Because of the areas of the burn, the nurse should be most concerned about the client developing laryngeal edema. Answer C would be the next priority. Answer A and B are incorrect because the client is mostly likely to experience the opposite conditions: hyponatremia and hypokalemia.

46. The client with hyperemesis gravidarum is at risk for developing which of the following conditions?

a. Metabolic acidosis with dehydration

b. Metabolic alkalosis with dehydration

c. Respiratory acidosis without dehydration

d. Respiratory alkalosis without dehydration

Answer A is correct. The client with hyperemesis gravidarum will have consistent nausea and vomiting which will cause dehydration. A dehydrated client will be in metabolic acidosis. Answer B is incorrect because a client who is persistently vomiting will not be in alkalosis. Answer C and D are both incorrect because the condition would be respiratory in nature.

47. The client who has just been in a motor vehicle accident is admitted to the emergency department. Findings reveal respirations 20, BP 80/34, and a pulse rate of 120. Which of the following nursing diagnoses should have priority?

a. Alteration in cerebral tissue perfusion

b. Alteration in sensory perception

c. Fluid volume deficit

d. Ineffective airway clearance

Answer C is correct. Checking for fluid deficit is the appropriate priority action in this case as the vital signs indicate the presence of hypovolemic shock. Answers A, B, and D are all incorrect because the findings do not indicate any alterations to the cerebral tissue perfusion, sensory perception, or an ineffective airway clearance.

48. The nurse is advising a client with recurring urinary tract infections. Which of the following diet instructions should the nurse give to the client?

a. Avoid citrus fruits

b. Drink a glass of cranberry juice daily

c. Increase intake of meats

d. Perform pericare with hydrogen peroxide

Answer B is correct. This is because cranberry juice is more alkaline and is excreted with acidic urine once it is metabolized by the body. Bacteria is less likely to grow in acidic urine and for this the client should be advised to drink cranberry juice on a daily basis. Answer A is incorrect because there is no need for the client to avoid citrus food. Answer C is incorrect because meat intake has no relation to urinary tract infections. And Answer D is also incorrect because although pericare should be performed, thus should not be done with hydrogen peroxide.

49. A client with preeclampsia and a blood pressure of 160/80, urinary output of 100ml for the last hour, and deep tendon reflexes 1+ has been admitted to the unit. The physician has ordered an infusion for magnesium sulfate. The nurse should:

a. Administer calcium gluconate and continue to monitor the blood pressure

b. Monitor the client's blood pressure but continue with the infusion of magnesium sulfate

c. Slow the infusion rate and turn the client on her left side

d. Stop the infusion of magnesium sulfate and contact the physician

Answer B is correct. The nurse should continue to assess the client's magnesium level and blood pressure and continue with the infusion. This is because both the client's blood pressure and urinary output are within normal limits. The only slight abnormalities are the deep tendon reflexes which are below the normal value. Answer A is incorrect because calcium gluconate is the antidote for magnesium sulfate. Answers C and D are also incorrect because there is no need to stop the infusion or to slow the infusion rate.

50. The LPN is reviewing the laboratory results of an 80-year-old client when she records a specific gravity of 1.020. The nurse evaluates that the client is experiencing which of the following?

a. A normal specific gravity

b. An impaired renal function

c. Diluted urine from fluid overload

d. Mild to moderate dehydration

Answer A is correct. The client with a specific gravity of 1.020 has normal specific gravity (the normal limits are from 1.010 to 1.025). Answers B, C, and D therefore incorrect.

51. A client with a hiatal hernia has been receiving magnesium hydroxide for relief of heartburn. The nurse should inform the client that overuse of magnesium-based antacids can cause which of the following?

a. Anorexia

b. Constipation

c. Diarrhea

d. Weight gain

Answer C is correct. An overuse of magnesium-containing antacids can lead to diarrhea. Answer A and D are incorrect because anorexia and weight gain is not associated with the use of magnesium antacids. Answer B is also incorrect because antacids containing calcium and aluminum cause constipation, and not those containing magnesium.

52. The nurse is caring for an obstetric client with dehydration. Which IV fluid should the nurse administer?

a. 45 normal saline

b. Dextrose 1% in water

c. Dextrose 5% in .45 normal saline

d. Lactated Ringer's

Answer A is correct. This is because normal saline is most like normal serum and is therefore the best IV fluid for the treatment of dehydration. Answers B, C, and D are incorrect because dextrose pulls fluid from the cell, dextrose with normal saline will alter the intracellular fluid, and lactated Ringer's contains more electrolytes than normal serum.

53. A client with urinary tract infection has an order for Pyridium (phenazopyridine hydrochloride). Which of the following should the nurse include in the teaching plan?

a. The medication ca cause changes in taste

b. The medication can cause diarrhea

c. The medication changes the color of her urine

d. The medication may cause mental confusion

Answer C is correct. Clients who have an order for Pyridium should be taught the drug will turn their urine orange or red. It can also cause yellowed skin. If taken in large doses, Pyridium can also cause a yellowish color to skin and sclera. Answer A, B, and D are all incorrect because the medication is not associated with changes in taste, diarrhea, or mental confusion.

54. A client receiving intravenous magnesium sulfate has been admitted to the unit. The nurse must closely observe for side effects associated with drug therapy. Which of the following is an expected side effect of magnesium sulfate?

a. Absence of knee jerk reflex

b. Decreased respirations

c. Decreased urinary output

d. Lethargy

Answer D is correct. Common side effects of magnesium sulfate include lethargy, hot flashes, and hypersomnolence. Answers A, B, and C are all incorrect because these are not common side effects of the medication.

55. The client informs the nurse that they have been experiencing diarrhea for the past three days. Which of the following acid/base imbalance would the nurse expect the client to have?

a. Metabolic acidosis

b. Metabolic alkalosis

c. Respiratory acidosis

d. Respiratory alkalosis

Answer A is correct. The client with persistent diarrhea is likely to develop metabolic acidosis due to the loss of bicarbonate (base). Answer B is incorrect because the alkalosis is caused by excess base (and not by a loss of bicarbonate base). Answers C and D are also incorrect because the condition relating to diarrhea is metabolic in nature, and not respiratory.

56. The nurse has been assigned to a client with a newly created ileostomy. When developing a care plan for the client, which of the following nursing diagnoses should be made a priority?

a. Deficient knowledge of ostomy care related to unfamiliarity with information resources

b. Disturbed body image related to presence of ostomy

c. Risk for deficient fluid volume associated to excessive fluid loss from ostomy

d. Risk for impaired skin integrity associated with the irritation from ostomy appliance

Answer C is correct. The diagnosis of risk for deficient fluid volume should be priority on the nursing care plan. Clients with a new ileostomy can experience high volume output of 1000–1800 mL per day when peristalsis returns. Because of this, the client's fluid intake needs to be increased to 2-3 liters a day. This fluid intake should include sports drinks in order to make up for lost sodium and potassium. Answers A, B, and D do apply to clients who have been diagnosed with ileostomy but they are not a priority in this situation.

57. An infant receiving intravenous fluid has been admitted to the unit. Which of the following indicates fluid overload in an infant?

a. Decreased blood pressure and decreased heart rate

b. Increased blood pressure and increased heart rate

c. Increased temperature and swelling of the feet

d. Increased temperature and swelling of the hands

Answer B is correct. Increased blood pressure and increased heart rate are both signs of fluid overload in an infant. Answer A is incorrect because A is the opposite of B. Answers C and D are also incorrect because the infant's temperature would not be increased by fluid overload.

58. Which of the following medications can potentiate a fluid volume deficit?

a. Inderal (propanolol)

b. Insulin

c. Lasix (furosemide)

d. Valium (diazepam)

Answer C is correct. This is because lasix is a non–potassium-sparing diuretic, which is a medication that can potentiate a fluid volume deficit. Answer A is incorrect because Inderal is a beta blocker which is used to treat cardiac disease and hypertension. It is not used to potentiate diuresis. Answer B is incorrect because insulin will not potentiate fluid volume deficit. Instead, insulin will force fluid back into the cell. Answer D is likewise incorrect because Valium, a phenothiazine, is utilized as an anti-anxiety medication and does not potentiate fluid volume deficit.

59. The client with isotonic dehydration is admitted to the hospital. The nurse can anticipate an order for which of the following IV fluids?

a. 3% sodium chloride

b. 45% sodium chloride

c. 5% dextrose and water

d. 9% sodium chloride

Answer D is correct. This is because the physician will order a fluid that contains normal saline to treat isotonic dehydration. Answer A is incorrect because this is a hypertonic solution. Answers B and C are also both incorrect because these are both hypotonic solutions.

60. The client with COPD is admitted to the unit. Findings reveal an oxygen saturation of 85%, a serum carbon-dioxide content level of 42 mEq/L, and a blood glucose level of 190 mg/dl. Upon evaluation of these findings, the nurse knows that the client requires which of the following?

a. A prescription for a bronchodilator

b. An injection of NPH insulin

c. Oxygen application with a venturi mask

d. Renal dialysis using an arterio-venous shunt

Answer A is correct. The client might need an order for a bronchodilator to help with the exhalation of carbon dioxide This is because the client's carbon dioxide content level is elevated (the normal serum carbon dioxide value is 24–30). Answers B and D are incorrect because the client's condition does not require an injection of NPH insulin or a renal dialysis. Answer C is likewise incorrect because oxygen should be administered via a nasal cannula and not with a venture mask.

61. The nurse infusing total parenteral nutrition (TPN) should also monitor intake and output carefully. What's the rationale for this?

a. To decrease the risk of fluid overload

b. To detect the development of hypovolemia

c. To determine the speed at which the client is metabolizing the solution

d. To determine whether the client's oral intake is sufficient

Answer B is correct. This is because common complications of TPN therapy include hypovolemia and osmotic. Answer A is incorrect because the risk of TPN therapy is hypovolemia and not hypervolemia. Answer C is incorrect because the client's intake and output would not reflect the metabolic rate. Answer D is likewise incorrect because the client will not usually be receiving oral fluids.

62. The doctor has prescribed 50mEq of potassium chloride for a client with a potassium level of 2.5mEq/L. How should the nurse administer this medication?

a. Continuous infusion over 24 hours

b. Continuous infusion over 30 minutes

c. Controlled infusion over five hours

d. Slow, continuous IV push over 10 minutes

Answer C is correct. When administering potassium chloride, an intravenous infusion controller should always be used. The maximum recommended rate of infusion for this drug 5–10mEq per hour. Intravenous infusion rate should never to exceed 20mEq per hour. Answer A is incorrect because the infusion time of 24+ hours is too long. Answer B is incorrect because the infusion time in this case is too short. Answer D is also incorrect because potassium chloride should never be administered IV push.

63. A client with renal calculi is admitted to the unit. Which of the following nursing interventions should be given priority?

a. Administering pain medication

b. Encouraging oral fluids

c. Initiating an intravenous infusion

d. Straining the urine

Answer C is correct. By increasing the client's fluid intake to 3,000mL every day, the client's urinary output will increase in frequency and volume. This will help prevent obstruction of urine flow from the kidneys and because of this, priority should be given to initiating intravenous fluids. Answer A is important but incorrect in this case because the administration of pain medication has no effect on preventing the obstruction of urine flow. Answer B is incorrect because the catheter is in the bladder and will therefore have no effect on the flow of urine from the kidney. Answer D is also incorrect because straining the urine will not help prevent the obstruction of urine flow (although it will help prevent some stones from developing).

64. The nurse has been assigned to a client who has just undergone abdominal cholecystectomy. The nurse is assessing the client's intake and output for the first 12 hours following the surgery. Which of the following findings should be reported to the doctor?

a. Absence of stool

b. Foley catheter output of 285mL

c. Nasogastric tube output of 150mL

d. Output of 10mL from the Jackson-Pratt drain

Answer B is correct. This is because the client's urinary output is below the normal value (the normal urinary output is 30–50mL per hour). This should immediately be reported to the doctor as it is a sign that the client requires additional fluids. Answer C is incorrect because for the first 12 hours following surgery, the client is not expected to have a stool. Answer C is incorrect because the output from the nasogastric tube is not excessive. Answer D is likewise incorrect because output from the Jackson-Pratt is expected to be small and therefore the finding is nothing out of the ordinary.

65. The nurse is caring for a client who is about to go into surgery. Which of the following laboratory findings should the nurse report to the doctor?

a. Blood glucose 75mg/dL

b. Hemoglobin 14.5g/dL

c. Potassium 2.5mEq/L

d. White cell count 8,000mm3

Answer C is correct. The normal potassium level is 3.5–5.5mEq/L. The nurse should therefore report to the doctor that the client's potassium levels are below the normal value. Answers A, C, and D are incorrect because all the given values are within the normal range.

66. The nurse is evaluating the laboratory results of a client's arterial blood gases. The PaCO2 indicates effective functioning of which of the following?

a. Kidneys

b. Liver

c. Lungs

d. Pancreas

Answer C is correct. PaCO2 stands for partial pressure of alveolar carbon dioxide and therefore signals the effectiveness of the lungs. Adequate flow of carbon dioxide is a major factor that contributes to acid-base balance in the body. Answers A, B, and D are all incorrect because their effectiveness is not signaled by PaCO2 findings.

67. The nurse is caring for a client with chest trauma client. Laboratory findings reveal a pH of 7.33, PCO2 55, PO2 85, and HCO3 27. The nurse evaluates the client as experiencing which of the following?

a. Compensated metabolic acidosis

b. Compensated respiratory acidosis

c. Uncompensated metabolic acidosis

d. Uncompensated respiratory acidosis

Answer B is correct. The blood gas results reflect the presence of respiratory acidosis. Both PCO2 and HCO3 are elevated (normal PCO2 is 35–45 and normal HCO3 with compensation is 22–26), and the pH value is decreased (normal 7.35–7.45). Answers A, C, and D are incorrect because these are not reflected in the laboratory findings given.

68. The nurse caring for an elderly client. Which of the following indicates to the nurse that the client has a fluid and electrolyte imbalance?

a. "I often feel thirsty"

b. "I regularly use a laxative for constipation"

c. "I sometimes have problems with dribbling urine"

d. "My always have dry skin"

Answer B is correct. This is because both the overuse and misuse of laxatives can lead to serious fluid and electrolyte imbalances in the elderly. Answer A is incorrect it has no relevance in this case. Answers C and D are both incorrect because these are normal occurrences associated with the changes that come from aging.

69. A client complains of exhaustion and muscle cramps after a running competition. Which of the following conditions would the nurse expect the client to be experiencing?

a. Hyperkalemia

b. Hypernatremia

c. Hypokalemia

d. Hyponatremia

Answer D is correct. This is because symptoms of hyponatremia include anorexia, exhaustion, muscle cramps, and an altered mental status. This is can arise in athletes who consume too much water when competing which can then result in decreased sodium levels. Answers A, B, and C are incorrect because they do not correlate with the symptoms given.

70. A client has been admitted to the burn unit 3 hours after sustaining second-degree burns to the trunk and head. Which of the following conditions would the nurse not expect to find during this time period?

a. Hyperkalemia

b. Hypernatremia

c. Hypovolemia

d. Laryngeal edema

Answer B is correct. This is because hypernatremia occurs when sodium moves out of the cell. This happens during the fluid shift phase of burn injury. Answers A, C, and D incorrect because they are more of a priority for this client.

71. The nurse checking a 40-year-old female client for hypovolemia. Which of the following findings would help the nurse in confirming a volume deficit?

a. BUN 18mg/dL

b. Hematocrit 55%

c. Potassium 5.0mEq/L

d. Urine specific gravity 1.016

Answer B is correct. Elevated hematocrit levels are a sign of hypovolemia. Answers A, C, and D are incorrect because the values given all within the normal level. The normal BUN value is 5–25mg/dL and the normal specific gravity value is 1.005–1.030, bot of which would be elevated with hypovolemia. Potassium levels can either increase or decrease with hypovolemia, the normal potassium level being 3.5–5.3mEq/L).

72. A client with a serum sodium level of 156mEq/L is admitted to the acute care unit. Which of the following should the nurse expect the client to exhibit?

a. Depression

b. Hyporeflexia

c. Manic behavior

d. Muscle cramps

Answer C is correct. The client has an elevated sodium level (the normal sodium level is between 135–145mEq/L) and is experiencing hypernatremia. Side effects of heightened sodium include mania and hyperactivity. Other symptoms of hypernatremia include seizures, restlessness, twitching, and hyperreflexia. Answers A and ad B are both incorrect because these are not signs of elevated sodium levels. Answer D is incorrect for the same reason and also because muscle cramp is a symptom associated with low sodium levels.

73. The client with metastatic cancer of the bone is exhibiting signs of mental confusion and a BP of 150/100. Which of the following findings would correlate with the client's symptoms as well as reflect a common complication that arises in clients with cancer of the bone?

a. Calcium 13mg/dL

b. Inorganic phosphorus 1.7mEq/L C

c. Potassium 5.2mEq/L A

d. Sodium 138mEq/L D

Answer A is correct. This is because hypercalcemia is a common complication in clients with metastatic cancer of the bone. Both mental confusion and an elevated blood pressure are symptoms of hypercalcemia. Answer B and D are incorrect because both values given are within the normal range. Answer C is incorrect because even though the potassium level given is elevated, it has no relation to the client's condition.

74. A client with increased intracranial pressure has been maintained on Furosemide (Lasix) and Osmitrol (Mannitol). The nurse knows that these two medications are given to reverse which effect?

a. Cellular edema

b. Energy failure

c. Excessive glutamate release

d. Excessive intracellular calcium

Answer A is correct. This is because the medications Lasix and Mannitol are administered for their diuretic effects in decreasing cerebral edema. Answers B, C, and

D are all incorrect because the drugs don't act to reverse energy failure, excessive glutamate release, or excessive intracellular calcium.

75. The client with a ruptured cerebral aneurysm has an order for Nimodipine (Nimotop). Which of the following is the intended effect of the medication?

a. Dissolve clotting that has formed

b. Prevent the inflammatory process

c. Prevent the influx of calcium into cells

d. Restore the client's blood pressure to normal

Answer C is correct. This is because Nimotop is a calcium channel blocker which is used to prevent calcium influx. Answers A, B, and D are incorrect because they do not describe the action of this medication.

76. A client admitted with a potassium level of 2.9mEq/dL and gastroenteritis has been placed on telemetry. Given the client's potassium results, which

of the following ECG findings should the nurse expect to see?

a. A depressed ST segment

b. A flattened QRS

c. An absent P wave

d. An elevated T wave

Answer A is correct. This is because depressed ST segments, peaked P waves, flat T waves, and high U waves are all ECG changes associated with low potassium levels. Answers B, C, and D are all incorrect because these are not ECG changes associated with hypokalemia.

77. The nurse is caring for a 24-hour post-burn client and notes the following laboratory values. Which of the these should the nurse immediately reported to the doctor?

a. Arterial pH 7.34

b. Hematocrit 52%

c. Potassium 7.5mEq/L

d. Sodium 131mEq/L

Answer C is correct. The client's potassium level is elevated (the normal potassium level is 3.5–5.0). The nurse must report this finding immediately to the doctor because complications which occur with hyperkalemia can be life-threatening. Answers A, B, and D are incorrect because the values given are all within the normal range.

78. The client who has just undergone abdominal surgery is having problems with his wound not healing up properly. Which of the following findings would most closely correlate with this problem?

a. Increased sodium

b. Increased calcium

c. Decreased creatinine

d. Decreased albumin

Answer D is correct. This is because protein plays a central role in wound healing and inadequate amount of protein would therefore correlate with the client's delayed healing of the wound. Answers A, B, and C are all incorrect because these values are not associated with wound healing.

79. A client with severe hematemesis is admitted to the medical-surgical unit. Which of the following nursing interventions should take priority?

a. Initiating an IV

b. Inserting an NG tube

c. Obtaining a blood permit

d. Performing an assessment

Answer D is correct. The first step the nurse should take is to assess the client for any signs or symptoms of fluid volume deficit. Answers Am B, and C are all interventions which are required later. They are incorrect because assessment is required before these other actions can be taken.

80. The nurse is caring for a client in the emergency unit. The nurse notices that it would contraindicated to induce vomiting if the client had ingested which of the following products?

a. Aspirin

b. Gasoline

c. Ibuprofen

d. Vitamins

Answer B is correct. This is because vomiting would be contraindicated with any petroleum, acid, or alkaline product. Answers A, C, and D are all incorrect because they do not contain any petroleum, acid or alkaline products.

81. The client with full thickness burns of both legs has been admitted to the hospital. The client's weight at admission was 182 pounds. Using the Parkland formula and the Rule of Nines, calculate the client's 24-hour intravenous fluid requirement.

Step-by-step answer:

Firstly, you will have to use the Rule of Nines to assess the percentage of burn:

Both legs of the client have been burned, each leg representing 18% TBSA. This makes a total of 36%.

The second step is to convert the client's weight into pounds. 185 pounds divided by 2.2 pounds = 84.09kg, which can be rounded up to 84 kg.

Lastly, you can estimate the amount of replacement fluid the client requires by using the Parkland burn formula:

(4 X 84 X 36) = 12,096 mL

Answer:

The client's 24-hour fluid requirement is 12,096 mL.

82. The nurse assessing the client for Trousseau's sign. The nurse is evaluating the client for which of the following conditions?

a. Hypocalcemia

b. Hypokalemia

c. Hypomagnesemia

d. Hyponatremia

Answer A is correct. A Trousseau's sign is evoked by placing a blood pressure cuff on the client's arm and inflating it to a pressure which is greater than the systolic blood pressure. If the client has hypocalcemia, he will be exhibiting visual manifestations of a positive Trousseau's sign; that is, twitches of the fingers, cramping, and spasms of the muscles of the hand and forearm which causes the hand and wrist to contract and flex down. Answers B, C, and D are incorrect because these conditions are not elicited by Trousseau's sign.

83. The nurse performing an assessment of a client with metabolic alkalosis. Which of the following findings should the nurse expect to observe in the client? Select all options that apply.

a. Circumoral paresthesia

b. Hypertonic muscle contractions

c. Kussmaul's respirations

d. Numbness of the extremities

e. Vomiting and nausea

f. Warm flushed skin

Answers A, B, and D are correct. Answers C, E, and F are all incorrect because these are symptoms of acidosis and not alkalosis.

84. Which of the following laboratory values should the nurse report to the doctor? Select all options that apply.

a. Calcium 12.0 mg/dL

b. Chloride 95 mEq/L

c. Magnesium of 2.6 mEq/L

d. Potassium 4.6 mEq/L

e. Sodium 90 mEq/L

Answers A and E are correct. Both these findings are abnormal. The normal level for Calcium is 8.5-10.5 mg/dL and the normal level of sodium is 135-145 mEq/L. Answers B, C, and D are all incorrect because the values given are all within the normal range and therefore don't need to be reported.

85. The nurse is caring for a client with pituitary tumor who has just undergone craniotomy. Which of the following laboratory values would make the nurse suspect a diabetes insipidus complication? Select all options that apply.

a. Hemoglobin of 13.6 g/dL

b. Low urine specific gravity

c. Normal serum chloride level

d. Serum potassium of 4.0 mEq/L

e. Serum sodium of 158 mEq/L

Answers B and E are correct. This is because clients with diabetes insipidus will exhibit an increase in urine output. Low specific gravity (< 1.005) in the urine and an increase in the sodium level (> 145 mEq/L) are therefore findings that can be associated with diabetes insipidus. Answers A, C, and D are all incorrect because the values give are within the normal range and because they have no relation to the disorder in this case.

86. The physician has ordered a calcium carbonate compound for a client in order to neutralize stomach acid. The nurse should monitor the client for which of the following?

a. Constipation

b. Diarrhea

c. Hyperphosphatemia

d. Hypomagnesemia

Answer A is correct. This is because constipation is a common side effect with clients who have been receiving calcium preparations. Answers B, C, and D are all incorrect because they are not associated with calcium carbonate intake.

87. A client with second-degree burns to the face, head, and trunk is admitted to the hospital two hours after the injury. Which of the following should the nurse be most concerned about?

a. Hyperkalemia

b. Hypernatremia

c. Hypovolemia

d. Laryngeal edema

Answer D is correct. Because of the area of the burn, the nurse should be most concerned about the client developing laryngeal edema. Answer C, hypovolemia, should be a second priority. Answers A and B are incorrect because these conditions are not of primary concern.

88. The nurse has been assigned to a client with adrenal insufficiency. Which of the following should take priority on the nurse's care plan?

a. Checking the client for signs of dehydration

b. Encouraging sleep and rest

c. Promoting a healthy body image

d. Providing high-calorie snacks

Answer A is correct. Clients with adrenal insufficiency will frequently exhibit acidosis and fluid volume deficit. Because of this, monitoring for signs of dehydration should therefore be a priority on the nurse's care plan. Answers B, C, and D are all incorrect because these options are not a priority.

89. A home health nurse is caring for a client congestive with heart failure who has been placed on diuretic therapy. Which of the following puts the client at risk of developing hypokalemia?

a. Midamor (amiloride hydrochloride)

b. Dyrenium (triamterene)

c. Demadex (torsemide)

d. Aldactone (spironolactone)

Answer C is correct. This is because Demadex is a loop diuretic and therefore depletes potassium. Answers A, B, and D are all incorrect because these drugs are all potassium-sparing diuretics.

90. A client with acute alcohol intoxication has been admitted to the unit and is receiving treatment for hypomagnesemia. Which of the following should the nurse expect to find during assessment?

a. A Positive Trousseau's sign

b. Bradycardia

c. Hypertension

d. Negative Chvostek's sign

Answer A is correct. This is because clients with hypomagnesemia will have a positive Trousseau's sign. Answer B is incorrect because the client would have tachycardia, not bradycardia. Answer C is incorrect because the client would have hypotension, not hypertension. Answer D is incorrect because the client would have a positive Chvostek's sign, not a negative one.

91. A client with gastroenteritis and dehydration has been admitted to the unit. The doctor has ordered intravenous fluid with potassium. Which of the following actions should the nurse take prior to adding potassium to the intravenous fluid?

a. Assess the client's urinary output

b. Obtain a stool culture

c. Obtain arterial blood gases

d. Perform a dextrostick

Answer A is correct. The nurse should check the client's urinary output before adding potassium to the intravenous fluid because during dehydration, the kidneys help to regulate any electrolyte imbalance by retaining potassium. Answer B and D are incorrect because they do not apply in this case. Answer C is incorrect because arterial blood gases measure respiratory compensation caused by dehydration.

92. The nurse is caring for a child diagnosed with cystic fibrosis. Which of the following findings taken from a sweat test supports the client's diagnosis?

a. A sweat chloride concentration greater than 60mEq/L

b. A sweat chloride concentration less than 40mEq/L

c. A sweat potassium concentration greater than 40mEq/L

d. A sweat potassium concentration less than 40mEq/L

Answer A is correct. This is because a child with cystic fibrosis will exhibit sweat concentrations of chloride which are greater than 60mEq/L. Answer B is incorrect a sweat concentration of chloride below 60mEq/L is too low to be diagnostic. Answers C and D are likewise incorrect because potassium concentrations are not used to make any diagnosis of cystic fibrosis.

93. The nurse is caring for a client with acute glomerulonephritis who is to be maintained on a low-potassium diet. Which of the following snacks is most suitable for the client?

a. Apple

b. Banana

c. Orange

d. Raisins

Answer A is correct. Apples are low in potassium and are therefore a good snack choice for clients who have been placed on a potassium-restricted diet. Answers B, C, and D are all incorrect because bananas, oranges, and raisins are all high in potassium.

94. The client with a sodium level of 100 mEq/L is admitted to the unit. Which of the following actions

should the nurse take after assessing the client's laboratory values?

a. Chart the finding

b. Contact the physician

c. Monitor the client's deep tendon reflexes for hypereflexia

d. Teach the client about low-sodium meal options

Answer B is incorrect. The nurse should contact the physician because the client's sodium level is below the normal range, which is 135–145 mEq/L. Answer A is incorrect because charting the laboratory values is not the correct action to take. Answer C is incorrect because assessing the client's deep tendon reflexes will not reveal hypereflexia. It is more likely to reveal hyporeflexia. Answer D is also incorrect because the client will need a diet that is high in sodium, not a low-sodium diet.

95. The nurse is assessing the client for a positive Trousseau's sign. Which of the following findings indicates a positive Trousseau's sign?

a. Abdominal tenderness

b. Carpopedal spasms

c. Facial grimacing

d. Nuchal rigidity

Answer B is correct. Twitching of the risk and muscular spasms are signs of a positive Trousseau's sign which in turn indicates that the client has hypocalcemia. Answer A and D are incorrect because abdominal tenderness and nuchal rigidity are not associated with the Trousseau's sign. Answer C is incorrect because facial grimacing is a sign of Chvostek's sign, and not Trousseau's sign.

96. The male client with hypercholesterolemia would like to know which vitamins can help him to lower his cholesterol. Which of the following has been seen to be effective in lowering cholesterol level?

a. Ascorbic acid

b. Cyanocobalamine

c. Niacin

d. Riboflavin

Answer C is correct. Niacin or B3 have both shown to be effective in lowering cholesterol levels. Answers A, B, and D are all incorrect because there is no data to show that these vitamins can facilitate lower cholesterol levels.

97. The nurse is caring for a 45-year-old client and is preparing to give an oral potassium supplement. How should the nurse administer potassium?

a. Without diluting it

b. With water only

c. With 4oz. of juice

d. On an empty stomach

Answer C is correct. To facilitate absorption and disguise the unpleasant taste of potassium, the nurse should always administer oral potassium supplements with at least 4oz of juice, ideally tomato juice. Answers A, B, and D are incorrect because all these options would cause gastric upset.

98. A client with periods of apnea has been admitted to the hospital after a closed head injury. The doctor has prescribed intubation and mechanical ventilation. Arterial blood gases reveal the following findings: a pH of 7.47, a HCO3 of 23, and a PCO2 of 28. The nurse assesses these findings as which of the following?

a. Metabolic acidosis

b. Metabolic alkalosis

c. Respiratory acidosis

d. Respiratory alkalosis

Answer D is correct. The client's blood gases reveal that the client is in respiratory alkalosis. Answers A, B, and C are therefore all incorrect because these conditions are not reflected by the values given.

99. The nurse has been assigned to a client with full thickness burns to the lower half of the torso and lower extremities. Which of the following is the primary nursing diagnosis during the emergent phase of injury?

a. A risk for fluid volume imbalance related to intracompartmental fluid shift

b. A risk for infection related to altered skin integrity

c. Acute pain related to burn injury

d. An imbalanced nutrition less than body requirements related to hypermetabolic state

Answer A is correct. This is because, during the emergent phase of injury, the nursing care priority for a client that has sustained burns to the lower body should be focused on the risk for fluid volume imbalance related to intracompartmental fluid shift. Answers B, C, and D are all incorrect because the risk for hypovolemia or fluid volume imbalance should take priority.

100. The client with intermittent confusion and a lack of mental alertness has been diagnosed with a fluid and electrolyte imbalance. Which of the following should be of primary concern to the nurse when caring for a client?

a. Risk of bleeding
b. Risk of dehydration
c. Risk of kidney damage
d. Risk of stroke

Answer B is correct. This is because the thirst mechanism declines with age. In elderly patient therefore, there is an increased risk of dehydration and high serum osmolality. Answer A, C and D are all incorrect because bleeding, kidney damage, or the risk of stroke are all not specifically related to fluid and electrolyte imbalances or aging.

101. The client with hypokalemia has been admitted to the unit. The nurse recognizes when assessing the client's history that the following medication could have contributed to the client's condition:

a. Corticosteroids
b. Muscle relaxers
c. Narcotics
d. Triamterene (Dyrenium)

Answer A is correct. This is because medications such as corticosteroids, amphotericin B, potassium-wasting diuretics, and large doses of certain antibiotics can cause excessive loss of potassium through the kidneys. Answer B and C are incorrect because muscle relaxers and narcotics do not typically affect the electrolyte and fluid balance. Answer D is also incorrect because Triamterene is a potassium-sparing diuretic which does not promote potassium excretion.

102. The client who has been maintained on spironolactone is exhibiting signs of EKG changes and muscle weakness. The nurse evaluates that the client is experiencing which of the following?

a. Hypercalcemia
b. Hyperkalemia
c. Hypocalcemia
d. Hypokalemia

Answer B is correct. This is because hyperkalemia can be caused by potassium-sparing diuretic such as spironolactone which acts to decrease potassium excretion in the body. EKG changes (peaked T waves, wide QRS complexes, and prolonged P-R intervals) and muscle weakness and twitching are all common symptoms of hyperkalemia. Answer A is incorrect because hypercalcemia has been associated with thiazide diuretics. Answer C is incorrect because hypocalcemia is not associated with the use of diuretic medications. Answer D is also incorrect because hypokalemia is seen in loop potassium diuretics such as furosemide (Lasix) or torsemide (demadex).

Study and Exam Preparation Tips

Studying for the NCLEX is a daunting challenge for every nursing student. Despite this, it is completely manageable and with the right approach, and success can be guaranteed.

In preparing for the NCLEX, there are three central elements that are of most important: **understanding, organization,** and **practice.** This study guide is designed for those who already have a good understanding of nursing practice. *Sections 2-6* of the guide are simply designed to refresh your memory and help you retain essential information that you will need to answer the practice questions in *Section 7.*

In this section, we have compiled some essential review strategies that will assist you in effective preparation for the NCLEX!

Study Tips:

- **Learning the details comes first!**
- Before going through the questions, it is important that you have come to grasp with the content that is being tested.

- Practice questions are designed to test and further your knowledge, and to make sure you know how to answer the questions efficiently and successfully.

- **Repetition is key!**
- Memorizing is key when it comes to dealing with conversion factors, laboratory values,

among other things. It is therefore useful to devote a set time each day to studying the information.

- On top of this, we encourage you to make best use of the time you spend commuting by continually going over key points.

- Repeating information just before you go to sleep also helps you memorize information you find particularly difficult to retain.

- **Test yourself!**
- As the old saying goes, practice is the key to success. The questions presented in this guide are representative of what you should expect in the NCLEX exam.

- Testing yourself is essential to knowing whether you are well prepared for the exam.

- Make sure to practice as much as possible and once you are getting closer to the actual exam, time yourself, allowing approximately one minute per question.

- **Learn from your mistakes!**
- If there are questions you haven't answered correctly, then see whether you understand the rationale and go over your revision notes again to make sure you have understood it fully.

- Make sure to test yourself again on questions that you initially answered incorrectly.

- All questions in this guide are numbered. Make sure to note down the questions you answered incorrectly and skip forward to these questions next time!

Exam Tips:

These are tips you should apply when you are sitting the exam. Try to also apply these when you are going over practice questions so it becomes second nature!

- **Read the questions carefully!**
- Being alert is key to successfully passing the NCLEX! Skimming through questions is the mistake most often made.

- It is crucial to make sure you read the question carefully and that you fully understand what it is the question is asking.

- If necessary, reword the question in your own words. This often helps in crafting an appropriate answer.

- **Look for keywords!**
- Keywords will help you work through the questions more efficiently.

- It is also advisable to avoid answers that include keywords such as all, always, every, except, must, never, no, none and only because they are rarely correct as they often limit or qualify the actual correct answer.

- **Use the method of elimination!**

- This is particularly useful if you are not straight away sure which option is the correct answer.

- Eliminate the answers that are clearly wrong, incorrect, or appear unfit until you cannot eliminate anymore.

- Another tip here is to look out for vague answers. Avoid vague answers and if you spot one, eliminate it!

- **The true-false test.**
- Treat each option as a true-false question and choose the option that is the 'most true'.

- **Trust your common sense!**
- Even if you're not 100% sure, knowing that you have studied rigorously and have gained a good knowledge of the content, it is often better to trust your instinct rather than risk running out of time.

- Even more than instinct, try and use your common sense and re-read the question again to see whether there is a key aspect you have overlooked at first sight!

- Another strategy that you can use is to read the question, answer the question and pick the option that most closely matches your answer.

- **Look for similar options.**
- Looking for the odd answer is a test strategy that can also prove very useful. See whether the three similar options are related to a

completely different topic and use the method of elimination or/and the true-false test to narrow down your correct answer.

- **Look for opposite/echo options.**
- If two questions are the opposite of one another, chances are that one of them is correct.

Final Notes

I would like to take this opportunity to thank you for purchasing this book. I hope you now have a solid foundation, and that this guide has helped you equip yourself with the knowledge for achieving success in the NCLEX, and throughout your nursing career.

My final piece of advice - no matter how diligent you are in your studies, your best learning will come from proactively practicing questions over and over again. I recommend revisiting the questions you have found difficult to constantly refresh and build on your knowledge as you progress.

I sincerely wish you the best of luck in your exam..
Best wishes,

Eva Regan